Single Best Answer &
Extended Matching Questions in

OBSTETRICS AND GYNECOLOGY

Single Best Answer & Extended Matching Questions in OBSTETRICS AND GYNECOLOGY

A Companion to Synopsis of Obstetrics and Gynecology

Justin C Konje
MBBS MD FMCOG (Nig) FWACS FRCOG MBA LLB PgCert Med Ed
Emeritus Professor
Department of Obstetrics and Gynecology
University of Leicester, UK
Senior Consultant, Feto-Maternal Medicine Centre
Doha, Qatar

Badreldeen I Ahmed
MBBS MD MBCHB FRCOG MFFP FAcadEd
Senior Consultant
Obstetrician and Gynecologist
Professor, Department of Obstetrics and Gynecology
Qatar University, Doha
Professor, Department of Obstetrics and Gynecology
Weill Cornell Medicine, Doha
Director, Feto-Maternal Medicine Centre
Doha, Qatar

JAYPEE

JAYPEE BROTHERS MEDICAL PUBLISHERS
The Health Sciences Publisher
New Delhi | London

JAYPEE **Jaypee Brothers Medical Publishers (P) Ltd**

Headquarters
EMCA House, 23/23-B
Ansari Road, Daryaganj
New Delhi 110 002, India
Landline: +91-11-23272143, +91-11-23272703
+91-11-23282021, +91-11-23245672
e-mail: jaypee@jaypeebrothers.com

Corporate Office
4838/24, Ansari Road, Daryaganj
New Delhi 110 002, India
Phone: +91-11-43574357
Fax: +91-11-43574314
e-mail: jaypee@jaypeebrothers.com

Overseas Office
JP Medical Ltd.
83, Victoria Street, London
SW1H 0HW (UK)
Phone: +44-20 3170 8910
e-mail: info@jpmedpub.com

EU GPSR Authorised Representative
Logos Europe, 9 rue Nicolas Poussin
17000, La Rochelle, France
Phone: +33 (0) 6 67 93 73 78
e-mail: contact@logoseurope.eu

Website: www.jaypeebrothers.com
Website: www.jaypeedigital.com

Inquiries for bulk sales may be solicited at: jaypee@jaypeebrothers.com

Single Best Answer & Extended Matching Questions in Obstetrics and Gynecology: A Companion to Synopsis of Obstetrics and Gynecology

First Edition: **2026**

ISBN: 978-93-6616-526-4

Printed in India at Sterling Graphics Pvt. Ltd.

Dedicated to

Our Late Parents

Titus Yangsi Kigha
Augustine Konje Tabe
Theresia Kien Tabe
Ibrahim Ahmed
Madina Suliman

Preface

Conscious of the rapidly changing world of medical knowledge driven by the information superhighway, and the need to have a synopsis that would allow easy learning enriched with illustrations, we produced this companion initially for medical students but as the writing evolved it became clear that we needed to produce a book that would be suitable for various grades of learning in the specialty.

The standards of the questions are such that about 50% would be suitable for undergraduates, another 25% for those sitting the Diploma in Obstetrics and Gynecology of the Royal College of Obstetricians and Gynaecologists, and most if not all of them suitable for various postgraduate examinations worldwide.

Extended matching questions are not only difficult to answer but equally difficult to set.

The questions in this book have been set following the layout of the Synopsis in Obstetrics and Gynecology. Each chapter in the synopsis is associated with a set of questions. Ideally, the two should be used in tandem; however, it should be easy to use either on its own.

We acknowledge that we have made every attempt to ensure that the contents of the questions are correct and up to date; however, we would first state that the answers and explanations are ours and thus there are undoubtedly occasions where we have misinterpreted the evidence, misread the question, or got it totally wrong. We would accept full responsibility for this and hope that candidates would be responsible enough to cross-check when there are doubts.

Justin C Konje
Badreldeen I Ahmed

Acknowledgments

We would like to express our gratitude to our families for their support and endurance while we were preparing the manuscript. We particularly thank Dr Mandy Abushama who not only bought into the project but also continued to give us advice and moral support. We would like to thank Mr Jovince for all the illustrations in the book. He was patient and tolerated our continuing revisions of the illustrations. Finally, we would like to thank M/s Jaypee Brothers Medical Publishers (P) Ltd, New Delhi, India, for taking on the task of publishing the book. The team has been very professional in their relationship with us.

Contents

SECTION A

Gynecology

PART A: Extended Matching Questions 1

- Basic Anatomy *1*
- Gynecology—History and Physical Examination *1*
- Puberty and Pubertal Disorders *2*
- Early Pregnancy Complications *3*
- Gynecological Oncology *15*
- Principles of Surgery in Gynecology *25*

PART A: Answer and Explanations.. 27

PART B: Single Best Answer Questions 40

- Basic Embryology *40*
- Basic Anatomy and Physiology of Reproduction *40*
- Gynecology History and Physical Examination *41*
- Puberty and Pubertal Disorders *41*
- Menstruation Physiology and Disorders of Menstruation *42*
- Early Pregnancy Complications *43*
- Gastrointestinal Disorders in Pregnancy (Constipation, Nausea, and Vomiting) *45*
- Puberty and Pubertal Disorders *45*
- Disorders of Menstruation or Abnormal Uterine Bleeding *46*
- Subfertility *48*
- Benign Conditions of the Uterus *49*
- Endometriosis and Chronic Pelvic Pain *50*
- Benign Ovarian Disorders *51*
- Sexually Transmitted Infections *52*
- Premalignant Disorders of the Genital Tract *54*
- Benign Conditions of the Vulva *54*
- Gynecological Oncology *55*
- Menopause and Hormone Replacement Therapy *59*
- Genital Prolapse and Urogynecology *61*
- Contraception *63*
- Principles of Surgery in Gynecology *65*
- Women's Health *67*

PART B: Answer and Explanations.. 68

SECTION B

Obstetrics

PART C: Extended Matching Questions 85

- Obstetric History and Examination 85
- Antenatal Care 85
- Normal Physiology of Pregnancy 86
- Fetal Growth and Monitoring 87
- Prenatal Diagnosis 89
- Multiple Pregnancy 91
- Bleeding in Pregnancy—Antepartum Hemorrhage 93
- Hypertensive Disorders of Pregnancy 94
- Diabetes and Endocrine Disorders of Pregnancy 97
- Other Endocrine Disorders of Pregnancy 99
- Dermatological Disorders of Pregnancy 99
- Respiratory Disorders of Pregnancy 100
- Connective Tissue Disorders of Pregnancy 102
- Cardiac Disorders in Pregnancy 102
- Renal Disorders of Pregnancy 103
- Infections in Pregnancy 104
- Psychiatric Disorders in Pregnancy 106
- Maternal Collapse in Pregnancy 107
- Intrauterine Fetal Death 108
- Preterm Labor and Premature Rupture of Fetal Membranes 109
- Hematological Disorders of Pregnancy 110
- Abdominal Pain in Pregnancy 112
- Induction of Labor 113
- Normal Labor 114
- Abnormal Labor 117
- Abnormal Presentation 119
- Operative Vaginal Delivery 120
- Episiotomy and Perineal Tears 121
- Postpartum Hemorrhage 122
- Puerperium and Puerperal Disorders 125
- Lactation 126
- Perinatal and Maternal Mortality 127
- Female Genital Mutilation 127
- Applied Genetics in Obstetrics and Gynecology 128

PART C: Answer and Explanations... 130

PART D: Single Best Answer Questions 156

- Obstetric History and Examination 156
- Antenatal Care 157

- Normal Physiology of Pregnancy *158*
- Fetal Growth and Monitoring *158*
- Prenatal Diagnosis and Management *160*
- Multiple Pregnancy *162*
- Bleeding in Pregnancy–Antepartum Hemorrhage *163*
- Hypertensive Disorders of Pregnancy *165*
- Diabetes and Endocrine Disorders of Pregnancy *166*
- Other Endocrine Disorders of Pregnancy *167*
- Dermatological Disorders of Pregnancy *167*
- Respiratory Disorders of Pregnancy *168*
- Connective Tissue Disorder of Pregnancy *169*
- Cardiac Disorders in Pregnancy *170*
- Renal Tract Disorders in Pregnancy *171*
- Infections in Pregnancy *172*
- Psychiatric Disorders in Pregnancy *175*
- Maternal Collapse in Pregnancy *176*
- Intrauterine Fetal Death *176*
- Preterm Labor and Premature Rupture of Fetal Membranes *177*
- Hematological Disorders of Pregnancy *179*
- Abdominal Pain in Pregnancy *181*
- Induction of Labor *182*
- Normal Labor *183*
- Abnormal Labor *186*
- Abnormal Presentation *187*
- Operative Vaginal Delivery *188*
- Episiotomy and Perineal Tears *189*
- Postpartum Hemorrhage *189*
- The Puerperium and Puerperal Disorders *191*
- Lactation *192*
- Perinatal Mortality and Maternal Mortality *194*
- Female Genital Mutilation *194*
- Fasting in Pregnancy *195*
- Applied Genetics in Obstetrics *196*

PART D: Answer and Explanations.. 197

Index...223

SECTION A

GYNECOLOGY

Part A: Extended Matching Questions

BASIC ANATOMY

Option list for questions 1–3

A	Anterior division of the internal iliac	F	Right ovarian vein
B	Columnar epithelium	G	Round ligament
C	Left ovarian vein	H	Transitional epithelium
D	Levator ani muscle	I	Transverse cervical (cardinal ligaments)
E	Posterior division of the internal iliac	J	Trigone

Instructions: Select from the option list above the anatomic structure that is described in each of the cases below. Each option may be chosen once, more than once, or not at all.

1. The uterine artery is the main supply to the uterus and originates from which structure within the pelvis?
2. Drains the left ovary directly into the renal vein, crossing over the vessels at the pelvic brim.
3. The main structure that supports the uterus from prolapsing.

GYNECOLOGY—HISTORY AND PHYSICAL EXAMINATION

Option list for questions 4–6

A	Cusco's speculum and bimanual examination	G	Lithotomy position
B	Cusco's speculum and endocervical and urethral swabs	H	Pap smear
C	Cusco's speculum and high and low vaginal swabs	I	Sims speculum
D	Dorsal position for inspection and bimanual examination	J	Transabdominal ultrasound scan
E	Magnetic resonance imaging (MRI)	K	Transvaginal ultrasound scan
F	Lateral position	L	

Instructions: These patients have attended the gynecology clinic with various complaints. You have taken a history and are about to undertake an examination and request for investigations. Choose from the list of options the best step you will next take in the management of each patient. Each option may be chosen once, more than once, or not at all.

4. A 16-year-old is seen in the clinic with a history of not yet menstruating. She has two sisters who started menstruating at the age of 12 years. She says that she has been having cyclical lower abdominal pain for the past 3 years. On palpation of the abdomen you suspect a mass in the left iliac region.
5. A 20-year old sexually active university student has been referred with a vaginal discharge and painful micturition for the past 4 days. She says that she has noticed a smelly discharge on her pants. She is on the combined contraceptive pill and is mildly tender on palpation of the abdomen.
6. A 56-year-old complaints of a lump in the vagina which is worse towards the end of the day but better when she gets up in the mornings. She says that she has to go to void more than before and also wakes up at night more than before.

PUBERTY AND PUBERTAL DISORDERS

Option list for questions 7–9

A	Androgen insensitivity syndrome (AIS)	**F**	Patau syndrome
B	Congenital adrenal hyperplasia (CAH)	**G**	Triploidy
C	Down syndrome	**H**	Turner mosaic
D	Edward syndrome	**I**	Turner syndrome
E	Klinefelter syndrome	**J**	

Instructions: The following girls presented with various abnormalities and following investigations including karyotype, various results were obtained. On the basis of the results, choose from the option list above which syndrome each girl has? Each option may be chosen once, more than once, or not at all.

7. A 15-year-old presented with primary amenorrhea and absent secondary sexual characteristics. She is examined and found to be 1.4 m tall, with widely spaced nipples, undeveloped breasts, a low hair line, and coarctation of the aorta on echography. A blood sample is sent for karyotyping and biochemistry. The result is high follicle-stimulating hormone (FSH) and luteinizing hormone (LH) and low 17-beta estradiol. The karyotype is reported as 45XO/46XX.
8. An 18-year-old sexually active student presents with primary amenorrhea. On examination, she is 1.65 m tall, with well-developed breasts but scanty pubic hair. Abdominal palpation shows bilateral inguinal hernias. The vaginal is short and ends blindly—no cervix. An ultrasound scan shows no uterus and no ovaries. Her karyotype is 46 XY and biochemistry shows raised FSH and LH as well as low 17-beta estradiol.

9. A newborn is diagnosed with ambiguous external genitalia. Urea and electrolytes show an electrolyte imbalance and the karyotype is 46XX.

EARLY PREGNANCY COMPLICATIONS

Option list for questions 10–12

A	Complete miscarriage	**F**	Incomplete molar pregnancy
B	Complete molar pregnancy	**G**	Missed miscarriage
C	Ectopic pregnancy	**H**	Recurrent miscarriage
D	Incomplete miscarriage	**I**	Septic miscarriage
E	Inevitable miscarriage	**J**	Threatened miscarriage

Instructions: Each of the women detailed below presented with complaints in early pregnancy. For each woman, choose from the option list above the single most likely diagnosis. Each option may be chosen once, more than once, or not at all.

10. A 26-year old presents with lower abdominal pains, bright red vaginal bleeding and amenorrhea of 8 weeks. She says she has passed blood clots and some liver-like tissues. A urine pregnancy test is positive. She is examined and is clinically stable with no abdominal pains. Vaginally, the bleeding has almost stopped. The cervical os is closed and the uterus is suspected to be normal in size.
11. A 19-year-old is admitted with excessive vomiting and a painless vaginal bleed. Her last menstrual period (LMP) was 10 weeks ago. A urine pregnancy test is positive. She is clinically stable and the uterus is about 16 weeks in size with no obvious fetal parts felt or heart sounds heard with a Sonicaid. At vaginal examination the cervix is closed and there are no adnexal masses.
12. A 22-year-old attends the emergency department with vaginal bleeding and abdominal pains at 9 weeks of gestation. She has passed some blood clots but no liver-like tissue. A urine pregnancy test is positive. There is no tenderness on abdominal palpation. On vaginal examination there are blood clots in the vagina and the cervical os is opened. A portable ultrasound shows a viable fetus in a regular gestational sac.

Option list for questions 13–15

A	Evacuation—surgical	**F**	Laparoscopic salpingectomy
B	Expectant management	**G**	Laparoscopic salpingostomy
C	hCG after 48 hours	**H**	
D	Methotrexate	**I**	
E	Misoprostol and mifepristone	**J**	

Instructions: Choose from the option list above the single most appropriate management that should be offered each of the patients presenting to the emergency with early pregnancy complications. Each option may be chosen once, more than once, or not at all.

13. A young girl has been admitted with vaginal bleeding that is associated with the passage of blood clots. The bleeding is continuing and she is complaining of severe lower abdominal pains. A urine pregnancy test is positive. Her LMP was 12 weeks ago. She is examined and found to have a blood pressure (BP) of 100/60 mm Hg and a pulse of 98 beats per minute. The abdomen is soft. On speculum examination, large blood clots are removed from the vaginal and active bleeding is coming from an opened cervical os. The uterus is about 10 weeks in size.
14. A young girl is seen in the Early Pregnancy Assessment Unit (EPAU) with left-sided mild abdominal pain and a brownish vaginal discharge. She is 6 weeks pregnant. A transvaginal ultrasound scan shows a 2 cm left unruptured tubal pregnancy with no fetal pole. The quantified hCG is 1,400 IU.
15. A woman who presents with disappearing symptoms of pregnancy is diagnosed with a missed miscarriage at 8 weeks of gestation. She had noticed that her breasts were no longer tender and the nausea and vomiting she had experienced earlier had stopped. She would prefer a treatment option that is be least invasive.

Option list for questions 16–18

A	Blood group	**G**	Speculum examination
B	Chest X-ray	**H**	Transabdominal ultrasound scan
C	Diagnostic laparoscopy	**I**	Transvaginal ultrasound scan
D	Full blood count (FBC)	**J**	Urinary β-hCG
E	Kleihauer test	**K**	Urine pregnancy test
F	Serum β-hCG		

Instructions: Choose from the option list above which test you would advise each of the women attending the EPAU to have following a clinical examination. Each option may be chosen once, more than once, or not at all.

16. A 20-year old presents with right-sided lower abdominal pain of 3 days duration. The pain is dull in nature. Her periods are irregular, but the last one was about 6 weeks ago. She has a positive pregnancy test and an ultrasound scan shows a thickened endometrium with no gestational sac and no adnexal masses or free fluid in the pelvis.
17. A woman is suspected to have an ectopic pregnancy. She presented after 6 weeks of amenorrhea with lower abdominal pains and a brownish

vaginal loss. She had an ectopic pregnancy a year ago that was treated by laparoscopic salpingectomy. A urine pregnancy test on admission was positive and serum β-hCG has been reported as 3,000 IU.

18. A 29-year-old was admitted with a threatened miscarriage at 10 weeks of gestation. She was stable on admission with minimal bleeding but had abdominal pains which is why she was admitted. She has suddenly collapsed and the bleeding is heavier. She is tachycardic and hypotensive.

Puberty and Pubertal Disorders

Option list for questions 19–21

A	Adrenal tumor	F	Hypothyroidism
B	Congenital adrenal hyperplasia	G	Iatrogenic drug induced
C	Constitutional	H	Neurofibromatosis
D	Cushing syndrome	I	Estrogen-producing ovarian tumor
E	Diabetes mellitus	J	

Instructions: For each of these young girls presenting with precocious puberty, select from the option list above the single most likely cause of the precocity. Each option may be chosen once, more than once, or not at all.

19. A 7 year-old presents with well developed breast, pubic, and axillary hair and menstruation which started 3 months ago. The mother says that she is slow, has been putting on weight, and struggles to cope with cold. When examined, she is found to be obese. A blood test is sent for biochemistry.
20. A 7-year-old presents with breast developed to stage 4 but no pubic or axillary hair. She does not have any other symptoms but says she has had some spotting vaginally.
21. An 8-year-old is seen in the clinic with well-developed secondary sexual characteristics and menstruation of 6 months duration. She does not have any other complaints. When examined, nothing abnormal is found.

Disorders of Menstruation or Abnormal Uterine Bleeding

Option list for questions 22 and 23

A	Adenomyosis	F	Malignancy
B	Coagulation disorder	G	Non-classified
C	Endometrial pathology	H	Ovulatory disorders such as in polycystic ovary syndrome (PCOS)
D	Iatrogenic	I	
E	Leiomyoma (fibroids)	J	

Instructions: These women present with abnormal uterine bleeding (AUB). For each woman choose from the list of options above the most likely cause of the AUB. Each option may be chosen once, more than once, or not at all.

22. A 27-year-old complaints of heavy menstrual bleeding associated with pains and painful sexual intercourse. She is examined and found to have a uniformly enlarged but not firm uterus that is tender on bimanual palpation and no adnexal masses.
23. A 33-year-old has been referred with irregular and heavy periods for the past 6 years. She says that her weight has been slowly increasing and she is also suffering from acne. Her body mass index (BMI) is 35 kg/m^2.

Option list for questions 24 and 25

A	Combined hormonal contraception	F	Myomectomy
B	Cyclical progestogens	G	Tranexamic acid
C	Hysterectomy	H	Uterine artery embolization
D	Levonorgestrel intrauterine system (IUS) (Mirena®)	I	
E	Mefenamic acid	J	

Instructions: Choose from the option list above the single best treatment for each of these women presenting with heavy menstrual bleeding. Each option may be chosen once, more than once, or not at all.

24. A 45-year-old has been suffering from heavy menses for more than a decade. She has had two blood transfusions because of this and was investigated and found to have uterine fibroids of approximately 20 weeks size. She is a mother of 3 and was sterilized 10 years ago. She is fit and well.
25. A 35-year-old mother of two presents with heavy menstrual bleeding. Her periods are regular but very heavy and she has to use superpads. She is taking iron tablets because of the heavy periods. Her partner uses the condom for contraception. When examined she is mildly pale and the uterus is normal in size with no adnexal masses.

Subfertility

Option list for questions 26–28

A	Anovulation—from PCOS	F	Klinefelter syndrome
B	Anovulation from hypogonadotropic hypogonadism	G	Mumps orchitis
C	Congenital absence of the vas	H	Sheehan's syndrome
D	Hyperprolactinemia	I	Tubal disease (from infections)
E	Intrauterine adhesions (Asherman syndrome)	J	

Instructions: Select from the option list above the single most likely cause of infertility in each of couples detailed below. Each option may be selected once, more than once, or not at all.

26. A couple are being investigated for secondary infertility. The woman had a baby 4 years ago. This was complicated by secondary postpartum hemorrhage for which she was treated with surgical evacuation. Her periods have never been the same since the surgery. They are very light—lasting for most times for just 1 day and only with spotting. They have, however, remained regular. Semen analysis on her husband has been normal.
27. A 26-year-old is being investigated for infertility after trying for 3 years. She has never been pregnant before and her periods are regular. She gives a history of right hypochondrial and lower abdominal pains a few years ago but says that these were never investigated as she subsequently got better. Her husband has no medical or surgical problems.
28. A couple with primary infertility is being investigated. The woman has regular cycles and no other problems. The man who has no significant past medical or surgical history has had two semen analysis and both have shown azoospermia. His hormone profile is normal.

Option list for questions 29–31

A	Chlamydia screening	**F**	Serum prolactin
B	Diagnostic laparoscopy and dye test—tubal patency test	**G**	Transvaginal ultrasound scan
C	Hysterosalpingography (HSG)—tubal patency test	**H**	21-day progesterone
D	Karyotype	**I**	
E	Semen analysis	**J**	

Instructions: Which most relevant investigation would you recommend for these patients who have been referred with infertility. Choose one option from the option list above. Each option may be chosen once, more than once, or not at all.

29. A couple has been trying for a baby for the past 18 months. The woman who weighs 60 kg is 28 years old and complaints in addition to a headache and a regular milky discharge from her breast. Her periods are irregular. The man is healthy and weighs 67 kg.
30. A couple has been trying for a baby for the past 2 years. The woman who is 26 years old has regular cycles and is healthy. The man who is 32 years old is also healthy. Their primary care physician has sent

some results of investigations which show that she is ovulating and the semen analysis on the man is normal. Both have also been tested for chlamydia infection and are negative.

31. A couple has been reviewed in the clinic with a 12 months history of primary infertility. The woman has regular cycles and her primary care physician performed a 21-day progesterone that was ovulatory. The man who is 40-year-old has no medical problems.

Benign Conditions of the Uterus

Option list for questions 32–34

A	Adenomyosis	F	Leiomyoma (fibroids)
B	Asherman syndrome	G	Nabothian follicles
C	Cervical ectropion	H	Pedunculated fibroid polyp
D	Cervicitis	I	
E	Endometrial polyp	J	

Instructions: On the basis of the clinical features and findings on examination, select from the list of options above the most likely diagnosis for each of these patients. Each option may be chosen once, more than once, or not at all.

32. A 30-year-old presents with intermenstrual bleeding, a copious clear vaginal discharge which is worse midcycle and postcoital bleeding. She is up to date with her cancer screening. Her periods are regular and the last one was 2 weeks ago. When examined there is a reddish cervix and nothing else abnormal.
33. A 27-year-old attends because her periods have become very light. She had an evacuation for retained products of conception following an incomplete miscarriage 6 months ago and since then her periods have become very scanty. She now menstruates for 2 days and does not have to wear a pad as its mainly in the form of spotting. There is no associated lower abdominal pain and the periods remain regular.
34. A 32-year-old complaint of painful periods for the past 6 years. The pain which starts a few days before her periods continues for about a week after. The periods are not heavy. She also has painful sexual intercourse especially after penetration. When examined, the lower genital tract is normal but the uterus is uniformly bulky and there are no adnexal masses.

Endometriosis and Chronic Pelvic Pain

Option list for questions 35–37

A	Acute pelvic inflammatory disease (PID)	**G**	Interstitial cystitis
B	Adenomyosis	**H**	Irritable bowel syndrome (IBS)
C	Adhesions	**I**	Ovarian cyst
D	Appendicitis	**J**	Primary dysmenorrhea
E	Chronic PID	**K**	Uterine fibroids
F	Endometriosis		

Instructions: The following patients are being reviewed in the clinic with the complaint of chronic pelvic pain (CPP). For each patient, use the information provided to suggest the single most likely cause of the clinical presentation. Each option may be chosen once, more than once, or not at all.

35. A 19-year-old says that she has been suffering from painful periods for the past 3 years. She started menstruating when she was 14 years old. The pain starts a day or two before her periods and is most painful on day 2 and 3 of her cycle. It then gets gradually better by the sixth to seventh day. Her periods usually last for 3–4 days. When examined there are no masses in the abdomen and the uterus was normal in size with mild bilateral adnexal tenderness.
36. A 36-year-old complaints of painful periods of 6 years. The pain which is mainly with menstruation lasts for 2–3 days and is associated with the passage of clots. She has had two normal deliveries—the last one was 8 years ago. When examined, the uterus is irregularly enlarged and firm in consistency. There are no adnexal masses and no tenderness on both sides.
37. A 20-year-old complained of severe pains with her periods and painful sexual intercourse. The pain is mainly during penetration. She says that her periods have always been painful. The pain which is spasmodic starts with menstruation and usually goes by the third day of her periods which are not heavy. She has been experiencing penetrative pain during sexual intercourse for the past 8 months. Using lubricants helps. When examined, nothing abnormal is found abdominally and on bimanual examination.

Option list for questions 38–40

A	Combined hormonal contraception	H	Medroxyprogesterone acetate (Provera)
B	GnRH agonist + Addback	I	Non-steroidal anti-inflammatory (NSAIDS)
C	GnRH antagonist + Addback	J	Ovarian cystectomy
D	GnRH agonist/estradiol/ norethindrone	K	Subcutaneous implant (Nexplanon)
E	Hysterectomy and bilateral salpingoophorectomy	L	
F	Laparoscopic excision or ablation	M	
G	Levonorgestrel intrauterine system		

Instructions: For each of the patients presenting with chronic pelvic pain, select from the option list above the best treatment you would recommend for the patient. Each option may be chosen once, more than once or not at all.

38. A 35-year-old mother of 3 comes to the clinic with chronic pelvic pain of 8 years duration. She has tried various oral hormonal options without success. She was sterilized a few years ago. She is examined and found to have a retroverted uterus with induration of the uterosacral ligaments and bilateral adnexal tenderness.
39. An ultrasound scan was performed on a 28-year-old who has been suffering from chronic pelvic pain and deep dyspareunia. The scan reports that there is a left ovarian mass measuring 6 × 7 cm and containing uniform fluid with bright speckles suggestive of hemorrhage. A diagnosis of an endometrioma is made.
40. A 19-year-old complaints of very painful periods for which she has to stay in bed for three days. The pains tend to last for 2–3 days and she says these have always been present since she had her first period. They are, however, getting worse and her periods which are regular are not heavy. She is not sexually active.

Benign Ovarian Disorders

Option list for questions 41–43

A	Brenner tumor	F	Hemorrhagic corpus luteum cyst
B	Dermoid ovarian cyst	G	Granulosa cell tumor
C	Endometrioma	H	Mucinous cystadenoma
D	Fibroma	I	Serous cystadenoma
E	Functional ovarian (follicular) cyst	J	Tubo-ovarian mass

Instructions: For each of the patients below, choose from the option list above the single most likely cause of her symptoms. Each option may be chosen once, more than once, or not at all.

41. A 7-year-old girl attends with her mother complaining of vaginal bleeding of sudden onset. The mother says that her breast started developing a few months ago. She however does not have any pubic or axillary hair. She has one sister who attained menarche at the age of 13 years. She is examined and found to have breast developed to Tanner stage 3 and no other secondary sexual characteristics. An ultrasound scan of the pelvis is performed and an ovarian cyst is found on the right ovary.
42. A laparoscopic ovarian cystectomy is performed on a 17-year-old who presented with an acute abdomen and a diagnosis of a torted ovarian cyst was made. At the laparoscopy she was found to have a right sided ovarian cyst that had twisted with the ovary and tube once around its pedicle. The ovary and tube were still pink hence it was untwisted and a cystectomy performed. The cyst ruptured and included in its contents was hair.
43. A 22-year-old has been referred because of pain which she developed a few days ago. The pain is mild and not associated with any systemic symptoms. Her primary care physician [general practitioner (GP)] had arranged an ultrasound scan which showed a 5 cm smooth-walled cyst on the right ovary with no echoes inside the cyst.

Sexually Transmitted Infections

Option list for questions 44 and 45

A	Candida albicans	F	Human immunodeficiency virus (HIV)
B	Bacterial vaginosis	G	Human papillomavirus (HPV)
C	*Chlamydia trachomatis*	H	*Neisseria gonorrhoeae*
D	Hepatitis B	I	Trichomonas vaginalis
E	Herpes simplex	J	

Instructions: Based on the clinical features described for each patient, choose from the list above the most likely diagnosis. Each option may be chosen once, more than one, or not at all.

44. A 19-year-old attended the genitourinary medicine clinic with a urethral discharge, right hypochondrial pain, and a low-grade fever. When examined, there is tenderness in the right hypochondrion and the lower abdomen with bilateral cervical motion tenderness.
45. A young girl comes to the emergency because she has not been able to void. She is examined and found to have widespread and extremely painful blisters on the vulva.

Option list for questions 46–48

A	Dark-field microscopy	F	Nucleic acid amplification test (NAAT)
B	Endocervical swab for culture and sensitivity	G	Nontreponemal test
C	Fourth-generation test	H	Treponemal test
D	Fluid for viral PCR	I	Wet preparation
E	Gram-negative stain	J	

Instructions: For each of the patients below, choose from the option list above the best test you will order to help make a quick diagnosis. Each option may be chosen once, more than once, or not at all.

46. You have seen a sexually active young girl who presents with a swollen and painful vulva, a discharge from the urethra, and pain passing urine. She also has pain in the lower abdomen. Her symptoms started 3 days ago.
47. A 30-year-old books for antenatal care in her first pregnancy. She is counseled and offered routine investigations. She indicates that she recently had a test for HIV which was negative.
48. The Emergency Doctor has seen a young girl with painful blisters on her vulva. The inguinal nodes are slightly tender and mildly swollen.

Option list for questions 49–51

A	Aciclovir	F	Combined retroviral treatment (cART)
B	Azithromycin	G	Doxycycline
C	Benzathine penicillin	H	Erythromycin
D	Ceftriaxone	I	Metronidazole
E	Ciprofloxacin	J	

Instructions: These patients have all be diagnosed with a sexually transmitted infection. Select from the list of options above the treatment of choice you would recommend for each infection. Each option may be chosen once, more than once or not at all.

49. A pregnant woman who books for antenatal care has just had a positive treponemal test after a positive non-treponemal test.
50. The diagnosis of genital herpes has been confirmed from viral PCR of vesiculate fluid aspirate from a 20-year-old who presented to the Genito-Urinary Medicine Clinic with painful vulval blisters.
51. A 38-year-old is seen in the Gynecology Emergency unit with painful micturition and a purulent discharge. There is associated lower abdominal pains. The vulva is red and tender posteriorly. NAAT is positive for *N. gonorrhoeae.*

Premalignant Disorders of the Genital Tract

Option list for questions 52–55

A	Back to routine recall screening (3–5 years)	F	Loop excision of the transformation zone
B	Colposcopy	G	Rescreen after 3 months
C	Cryotherapy	H	Rescreen after 6 months
D	Directed biopsy	I	Rescreen after 12 months
E	HPV test of cure after 6 months	J	
F	HPV triage and cytology		
G	Hysterectomy		

Instructions: For each of the women detailed below who has attended for cervical cancer screening, select from the list of options above the single most appropriate action in response to the result of the screening. Each option may be chosen once, more than once, or not at all.

52. A woman attends for a routine cervical cancer screen and the report is high-risk HPV (HR-HPV) positive and cytology is normal.
53. The screen result of a 45-year-old has been reported as HR-HPV positive and borderline cytology.
54. A patient who had HR-HPV positive and an abnormal cytology had colposcopy and was treated by large loop excision of the transformation zone (LLETZ).
55. The screen test was HR-HPV positive and a negative cytology initially. 12 months later this has been reported as HR-HPV negative.

Benign Conditions of the Vulva

Option list for questions 56–58

A	*Candida albicans*	F	Lichen sclerosus
B	Dermatitis (vulva eczema)	G	Paget's disease
C	Herpes simplex	H	Psoriasis
D	HPV	I	Vulvodynia
E	Lichen planus	J	

Instructions: These women all present with symptoms of benign vulva disorders. For each woman, choose from the option list above the most likely cause of her symptoms. Each option may be chosen once, more than once, or not at all.

56. A 65-year-old postmenopausal woman complaints of itching in the vulva of 6 months duration. There is associated soreness which started

with scratching. Sexual intercourse has become very painful and she is now avoiding her husband. When examined the labia appear pale and thin with the minora fused in the midline.

57. A 45-year-old visits her GP complaining of itching and soreness of the vulva. She dates this to a holiday abroad where she spent time on the beach and used a special cream to avoid sunburn. There is no associated vaginal discharge. The vulva appears red, with areas of hyperpigmentation and fissuring.
58. A 50-year-old teacher visits the doctor complaining of a burning pain in the vulva of 6 months duration. She does not have any vaginal discharge but is unable to allow her husband to come near her because of pain. When examined, the vulva appears normal but on touching she jumps from severe pain.

Option list for questions 59–61

A	Bacterial vaginosis	F	*Streptococcus pyogenes*
B	*Chlamydia trachomatis*	G	*Trichomonas vaginalis*
C	*Gardnerella vaginalis*	H	*Vulvovaginal candidiasis*
D	*Haemophilus influenzae*	I	
E	*Neisseria gonorrhoeae*	J	

Instructions: For each of the patients coming to the clinic with symptoms of an infection in the genital tract, select from the option list above the single most likely cause of the infection. Each option may be selected once, more than once, or not at all.

59. The symptoms this patient presented with included a thin offensive and sometimes fishy odorous vaginal discharge and soreness. When examined the vagina is coated with a discharge but neither the vulva nor vagina are inflamed. The pH of the vaginal discharge is 5.2 and microscopy shows clue cells.
60. The patient, a 26-year-old Police Officer, presented with a profuse offensive vaginal discharge which is frothy and yellowish/greenish in color. She has some itching in the vulva. The vulva appears slightly red and the vagina is inflamed. The appearance of the cervix is strawberry-like and the pH of the vagina is measured as 5.6.
61. The 30-year-old presents with recurrent vaginal discharge for 18 months. She has type II diabetes for which she is taking metformin (Glucophage). The discharge which is on and off is thick and whitish but nonoffensive. She also complaints of itching of the vulva. The vulva is red and swollen and there is a cheese-like discharge on the vaginal walls. The pH of the vagina is 4.0.

GYNECOLOGICAL ONCOLOGY

Option list for questions 62–64

A	Chemoradiation	F	Radical hysterectomy (Wertheim's hysterectomy
B	Chemotherapy	G	Simple hysterectomy
C	Cone biopsy	H	Trachelectomy
D	External radiotherapy and brachytherapy (intracavitary)	I	
E	LLETZ	J	

Instructions: These patients present with clinical features of cervical cancer. For each patient choose from the option list above the single most appropriate treatment. Each option may be chosen once, more than once, or not at all.

62. A 32-year-old who has never been pregnant attends for her routine cervical cancer screening. She is HR-HPV positive and therefore had a colposcopy. At colposcopy a suspicious area is identified on the cervix and a biopsy confirms this to be microinvasive cervical cancer (stromal invasion is <3 mm). She recently got married and is also trying for a baby.
63. A 42-year-old mother of 2 who presented with postcoital bleeding and a vaginal discharge has been examined and there is a suspected lesion on the cervix that measures about 2 × 2 cm. It is biopsied and the histology report comes back as cervical cancer. An MRI is performed and shows spread to the parametrium. At examination under anesthesia she was staged as IIA.
64. A 45-year-old who was diagnosed with cervical cancer from a punch biopsy undergoes an examination under anesthesia and MRI and the cancer is staged as IIB.

Option list for questions 65–67

A	Stage 1A1	H	Stage IIB
B	Stage 1A2	I	Stage IIIA
C	Stage 1B1	J	Stage IIIB
D	Stage IB2	K	Stage IIIC
E	Stage IB3	L	Stage IVA
F	Stage IIA1	M	Stage IVB
G	Stage IIA2		

Instructions: Choose from the list of options above the single most suitable stage of cancer for each of the patients detailed below. Each option may be chosen once, more than once, or not at all.

65. A 38-year-old presented with irregular vaginal bleeding and a brownish discharge. She is examined and found to have an exophytic lesion on the cervix which has been confirmed as well-differentiated squamous cervical cancer on histology with stromal invasion of 2 cm. An MRI does not show any spread to the parametrium. An examination under anesthesia (EUA) is performed and the upper two-thirds of the vagina is involved and the parametrium and pelvic side wall are not involved.
66. At EUA for staging of cervical cancer in a 50-year-old patient, she is found to have spread to the pelvic side wall, to the upper vagina but no involvement of the bladder or rectum. An ultrasound scan performed prior to the EUA had shown a right hydroureter. An MRI does not show any pelvic node involvement.
67. A colposcopy was performed on a 32-year-old who had attended with a persistent vaginal discharge and postcoital bleeding. A suspected area on the squamocolumnar junction was biopsied and shown to be squamous carcinoma that had invaded the stroma by 1.5 mm.

Endometrial Cancer

Option list for questions 68–70

A	Clear cell carcinoma	**F**	Sarcoma of the myometrium
B	Endocrine carcinoma	**G**	Serous carcinoma of the uterus
C	Endometrial hyperplasia with atypia	**H**	Well-differentiated adenocarcinoma
D	Endometrial hyperplasia without atypia	**I**	
E	Mixed carcinoma	**J**	

Instructions: The following are treatment methods for pathologies of the endometrium or uterus. For each treatment, choose from the option list the type of pathology for which it will be the treatment of choice. Each option may be chosen once, more than once, or not at all.

68. A 40-year-old with irregular periods whose endometrial biopsy has come back and following review was placed on oral progestogens.
69. A 36-year-old who was diagnosed with PCOS when she was 25 years now complaints of very infrequent but heavy periods. She had an endometrial biopsy and was offered treatment but wishes to have children first.
70. A 60-year-old who presented with postmenopausal bleeding and following investigations was offered a total laparoscopic abdominal hysterectomy and BSO as an urgent procedure.

Option list for questions 71–73

A	Stage 1A	F	Stage IIIC1
B	Stage 1B	G	Stage IIIC2
C	Stage II	H	Stage IVA
D	Stage IIIA	I	Stage IVB
E	Stage IIIB	J	

Instructions: Based on the description of the extent of cancer in the patients below, choose from the option list the stage that best describes the cancer. Each option may be chosen once, more than once, or not at all.

71. A hysterectomy is performed on a woman who presented with postmenopausal bleeding. The histology report concludes that she has well differentiated carcinoma with vascular permeation and invading about 20% of the myometrium.
72. The histology on specimens removed at surgery from a patient who was diagnosed with endometrial carcinoma from a Pipelle biopsy shows carcinoma of the endometrium that invades the cervical stroma but does not extend beyond the uterus.
73. The tumor has invaded the bladder but there are no distant metastases.

Ovarian and Fallopian Tube Cancer

Option list for questions 74–76

A	Dysgerminoma	F	Mucinous cystadenocarcinoma
B	Endodermal sinus tumor	G	Serous cystadenocarcinoma
C	Endometrioid cystadenocarcinoma	H	Sertoli–Leydig tumor
D	Granulosa cell tumor	I	
E	Immature teratoma	J	

Instructions: For each of the patients below choose from the option list above the single most likely type of ovarian tumor. Each option may be selected once, more than once, or not at all.

74. A 69-year-old woman who presented with postmenopausal bleeding was found on ultrasound scan to have an ovarian tumor. Tumor markers were measured and inhibin was found to be raised.
75. A 65-year-old presents with vague abdominal pains and swelling of 6 months duration. An ultrasound scan shows a complex ovarian cyst with solid and cystic areas and some ascites. CA125 is raised (378 U/mL) (normal 0–35 U/mL). She reports that her mother had cancer of the ovary at the age of 56 years.

76. A 45-year-old complaints of hirsutism, deepening voice, and amenorrhea of 3 months duration. When examined there is a left-sided ovarian mass which is confirmed on ultrasound scan.

Option list for questions 77–79

A	Stage 1A	H	Stage IIIA1
B	Stage 1B	I	Stage IIIA2
C	Stage 1C1	J	Stage IIIB
D	Stage 1C2	K	Stage IIIC
E	Stage 1C3	L	Stage IVA
F	Stage IIA	M	Stage IVB
G	Stage IIB	N	

Instructions: All these patients have been diagnosed with ovarian cancer. Choose from the option list above the stage of ovarian cancer that best applies to each patient. Each option may be chosen once, more than once or not at all.

77. The patient had surgery for an ovarian tumor and was found to have a serous cystadenocarcinoma confined to one ovary with an intact capsule and no malignant cells in ascitic fluid or peritoneal washings.
78. The patient had an ovarian cyst which ruptured during surgery. Histology of the cyst shows it to be a serous cystadenocarcinoma with no malignant cells in ascitic or peritoneal washings.
79. Staging laparotomy shows a large left ovarian complex tumor with seedlings on the bowel and omentum, some of which measured about 2 cm. There are no tumors in the retroperitoneal nodes or beyond the abdomen.

Vulva and Vaginal Cancer

Option list for questions 80–82

A	Stage Ia	G	Stage IBIb(ii)
B	Stage Ib	H	Stage IIIc
C	Stage II	I	Stage IV(i)
D	Stage IIIa(i)	J	Stage IV(ii)
E	Stage IIIa(ii)	K	Stage IVb
F	Stage IIIb(i)	L	

Instructions: For each of these women with a diagnosis of cancer of the vulva, choose from the option list the best description of the stage of the disease. Each option may be chosen once, more than once, or not at all.

80. A 60-year-old presented with an ulcer on her right vulva. When examined this was located on the labium majorum and about 3 cm from the midline. It measured 1.5 cm in its maximum diameter and there were no associated nodes. An MRI was negative for node involvement or local spread. A biopsy showed no invasion of the surrounding tissues.
81. A 73-year-old who presented with a bleeding ulcer on vulva was examined and found to have a suspicious looking ulcer that measured 3 cm on the left labium majorum. There was a suspicion that the lesion had invaded the lower vagina but there were no palpably enlarged nodes. An MRI confirmed that there was no lymphadenopathy. A biopsy revealed a well differentiated squamous cell carcinoma that had invaded the lower third of the vagina.
82. A 70-year-old retired teacher presents with a lump on her vulva with associated itching but no bleeding. She is examined and found to have a pigmented lesion on the right vulva about 1 cm from the midline posteriorly. There is an ulcer on the pubic symphysis with associated enlarged inguinofemoral nodes. An MRI of the abdomen and pelvis shows enlarged nodes and secondaries in the liver. A chest X-ray shows no lesions in the lungs. A biopsy confirms these lesions to be cancer.

Option list for questions 83–85

A	Biopsy for histology	G	MRI of the pelvis and abdomen
B	Cervical cytology	H	Positron emission tomography (PET) scan
C	Chest X-ray	I	Ultrasound scan of the pelvis
D	Colposcopy	J	
E	EUA	K	
F	FBC and live function test	L	

Instructions: These patients present with lesions on their vulva or vagina. For each patient select from the option list the most useful investigation to perform at this stage of her management. Each option may be chosen once, more than once, or not at all.

83. A postmenopausal woman presents with itching of the vulva and soreness of 6 months duration. She has been examined and there is a raised lesion on the mons pubis which is hard and measures 2.3 cm which is hyperpigmented. The inguinal lymph nodes are enlarged. Vulva cancer is suspected.
84. A woman in her 70s has been diagnosed with vaginal carcinoma from a biopsy of an ulcer on the vaginal wall. Clinical examination at the time of the biopsy had shown a 2.2 cm ulcer on the lateral vaginal wall about 3 cm from the introitus.

85. A 64-year-old had wide excision and ipsilateral lymphadenectomy for left vulva carcinoma. The histology report showed free lateral margins and tumor involvements of three lymph nodes. She is now coming for follow-up.

Option list for questions 86–88

A	Adjuvant radiotherapy	**H**	Radical hysterectomy and vaginectomy
B	Adjuvant chemotherapy	**I**	Radical wide excision and bilateral groin dissection
C	Chemotherapy	**J**	Radical wide excision and ipsilateral lymph node dissection
D	Chemoradiation	**K**	Radiotherapy
E	Neoadjuvant chemotherapy	**L**	Total vaginectomy
F	Palliative care	**M**	
G	Radical vulvectomy	**N**	

Instructions: For each of these women with a diagnosis of cancer of the vulva, choose from the option list above the single most appropriate treatment option. Each option may be chosen once, more than once, or not at all.

86. A 60-year-old woman has been diagnosed with squamous cell carcinoma of the vulva that is located 3 cm from the midline with no associated lymphadenopathy. An MRI showed no local spread of the disease. She is fit and has a normal FBC and LFT.
87. Radical excision and bilateral groin node dissection was performed on a 58-year-old women with vulva cancer. The histology report shows a 5 mm free margin and 3 positive nodes.
88. A 70-year-old has been diagnosed with carcinoma of the vagina stage II. She is fit and well.

Option list for questions 89 and 90

A	Stage Ia	**G**	Stage IVb
B	Stage Ib	**H**	
C	Stage IIa	**I**	
D	Stage IIb	**J**	
E	Stage III	**K**	
F	Stage IVa	**L**	

Instructions: Each of the patients detailed below have been diagnosed with cancer of the vagina. Choose from the option list above the single best stage of the cancer. Each option may be chosen once, more than once, or not at all.

89. A 79-year-old presents with postmenopausal bleeding for the past 6 weeks. She is examined and found to have a suspicious looking area measuring 1 × 1 cm on the left lateral vagina wall (about 4 cm from the introitus). This is biopsied and histologically shown to be squamous carcinoma of the vagina confined to the vaginal wall. An MRI of the pelvis does not show any spread beyond the vagina wall and no lymph node involvement.
90. The woman who is 80 years old complaints of a vaginal discharge with occasional blood stain of 6 months duration. There has been associated lower back and pelvic pain which is getting worse. When examined, there is a suspicious lesion on the posterior anterior lower third of the vaginal wall. The paravaginal tissue appears involved. An MRI shows left hydronephrosis and enlarged lymph nodes.

Menopause and Hormone Replacement Therapy

Option list for questions 91–93

A	Acupuncture	G	Moisturizers
B	Combined estrogen and progestogens	H	Estrogen tablets
C	Combined estrogen and progestogen and testosterone implants	I	Progestogen tablets
D	Fluoxetine	J	Reflexology
E	Hypnotism	K	
F	Lifestyle and dietary modifications		

Instructions: These women present with menopausal symptoms. For each woman, choose from the option list above the best recommendation for her menopausal symptoms. Each option may be selected once, more than once, or not at all.

91. A 56-year-old who had a hysterectomy and BSO 8 years ago attends with vaginal dryness and superficial dyspareunia. She is otherwise well although she has occasional night sweats and hot flushes.
92. A 55-year-old teacher complaints of mood swings night sweats, hot flushes, and loss of interest in sex because of superficial dyspareunia. She has tried various nonmedical options recommended by her GP unsuccessfully. Her BP is normal and there is nothing of significance in her past or current medical history. Her BMI is 28 kg/m^2.
93. A 50-year-old attends with severe hot flushes and night sweats of 6 months duration. Her periods are now irregular and very infrequent—the last one was 3 months ago. She is hypertensive on treatment with labetalol 200 mg BD and also diabetic on metformin. Her BMI is 34 kg/m^2.

Genital Prolapse and Urogynecology

Option list for questions 94–96

A	Ambulatory urodynamics	F	Ultrasound scan of the bladder, kidneys, and ureters
B	Bladder scan	G	Urea and electrolytes
C	Cystoscopy	H	Urinalysis
D	Pad test	I	Urodynamics
E	3-day voiding diary	J	

Instructions: These patients present with symptoms of urinary incontinence. For each patient, choose from the list of options above the best initial investigation you will recommend for the patient. Each option may be selected once, more than once, or not at all.

94. A 48-year-old comes to the clinic complaining of frequency, urgency, and urge incontinence. She also says that she has a dragging sensation in the vagina which is worse at the end of the day. Because of the frequency and urge incontinence she has become frightened of going out as she is afraid to embarrass herself in public.
95. A 50-year-old physical education teacher complaints that she struggles to remain dry during exercises with her students. Every time she jumps she wets herself. These symptoms which started 9 months ago have been getting worse. She does not pass urine more often than before and does not feel the urge to go or wet herself when she feels like going. She does not have any pressure symptoms in the vagina and rarely gets up at night to void. Her GP has tested her urine and excluded an infection.
96. A 37-year-old had a normal vaginal delivery 3 months ago and since then has been struggling with her waterworks. She voids more often than normal and leaks sometimes uncontrollably. She had an epidural for labor and her symptoms started shortly after. She has been investigated for urine infections on many occasions, and these have always been negative.

Option list for questions 97–99

A	Bladder overflow with incontinence	F	Urinary fistula
B	Low compliance bladder	G	Urodynamic stress incontinence
C	Mixed urinary incontinence	H	
D	Outflow obstruction	I	
E	Overactive bladder	J	

Instructions: For each of these patients presenting with symptoms of urinary incontinence, select from the option list above the most likely diagnosis. Each option may be chosen once, more than once, or not at all.

97. A 58-year-old complaints of stress urinary incontinence, frequency, urgency, and urge incontinence of 2 years duration. At the beginning it was mainly incontinence when she sneezed or coughed, but now if she does not rush when she feels like going, she will wet herself. She has increasingly been going to empty her bladder more often than before although she does not drink more than usual.
98. A 43-year-old Nursing Sister reports that she has been unable to control her urine for the past 12 months. She is a mother of two—all normal vaginal deliveries. The symptoms are mainly with sneezing and lifting, especially when she has to lift patients on the ward. Her fluid intake has not changed and she does not feel any lump or dragging sensation in the vagina. She also does not wake up at night to void. When examined, she is obese (BMI—33 kg/m^2) but there are no signs of genital prolapse.
99. A 69-year-old retired Council Clerk complaints of urinary incontinence of 3 yeas duration. This has progressively got worse to the extent that she now rarely goes out. She has to go almost every 1–2 hours so as to avoid wetting herself. When she feels like going, she has to rush. She voids small volumes and over the last 6 months has been sleeping very poorly as she has to wake up many times to void. There are no symptoms of prolapse.

Option list for questions 100–102

A	Anterior repair	**F**	Duloxetine
B	Anticholinergics	**G**	Pelvic floor exercises
C	Bladder retraining	**H**	Sling operation [e.g., transvaginal tape (TVT)]
D	Botulinum toxin	**I**	Topical estrogens
E	Colposuspension	**J**	

Instructions: Choose from the option list above the best first-line treatment you will offer each of the women below. Each option may be chosen once, more than once, or not at all.

100. This is a 38-year-old who has been diagnosed with urodynamic stress incontinence and no other problems.
101. The patient is a 56-year-old who complaints of urinary frequency and incontinence associated with urgency and urge incontinence. A 3-day voiding diary and urodynamics has diagnosed an overactive bladder.
102. A 61-year-old was diagnosed with an overactive bladder and offered pelvic floor exercises and bladder retraining. She now attends after 6 months with no improvements in her symptoms.

Option list for questions 103–105

A	Anterior repair	F	Sacrocolpopexy
B	Anterior vaginal and perineal repair	G	Sacrospinous fixation
C	Colpocleisis	H	Shelf pessary
D	Posterior repair	I	Vaginal hysterectomy
E	Ring pessary	J	Vaginal hysterectomy and repair

Instructions: These women present with symptoms of urogenital prolapse. For each woman, choose the most appropriate treatment you would recommend from the option list above. Each option may be chosen once, more than once, or not at all.

103. A 60-year-old who presented with a dragging sensation in the vagina and no associated urinary symptoms is found on examination to have a prolapse of the lower posterior vaginal compartment. The uterus which is atrophic does not descend beyond the ischial spines.
104. A 65-year-old is seen with an 18 months history of a lump in her vagina. This has been gradually getting worse and now she has to push it back to completely empty her bladder. She is sexually active but finds it embarrassing so avoids her husband as much as possible. She has been experiencing an increase in frequency of micturition but no incontinence. She is examined and found to have a large prolapse of the anterior vaginal wall and the cervix is just below the ischial spines.
105. An 88-year-old frail woman has been referred because of genital prolapse. She has a lump outside the vagina which is very uncomfortable. She says that this started about 8 years ago and has gradually got worse. At the outset it was just a dragging sensation but with time a lump appeared but then disappeared when she went to sleep but over the last 2–3 years it has not been going back. When examined the whole of an atrophic uterus is outside the introitus. She is hypertensive and suffers from chronic obstructive airway disease.

Contraception

Option list for questions 106–109

A	Combined hormonal patch	G	Minipill (progestogen only tablets)
B	Combined contraceptive pills	H	Levonorgestrel IUS (Mirena®)
C	Combined hormonal contraceptive ring	I	Sterilization—female
D	Copper intrauterine device (IUD)	J	Sterilization—male
E	Depo-Provera	K	Subdermal implant (Nexplanon)
F	Lactational amenorrhea (LAM)	L	

Instructions: Choose from the option list above the best form of contraception for each of the women who is presenting below. Each option may be chosen once, more than once, or not at all.

106. A 20-year-old has just had an abortion and wishes to go on an effective contraceptive. Her periods are regular. Her BMI is 24 kg/m^2. Her periods are painful and the pain is mainly from day 1 to 6 of the cycle. She is not very keen to take regular medication.
107. A 27-year-old who is known to suffer from oligomenorrhoea, weight gain, acne, and hirsutism wishes to go on an effective contraceptive. Her BMI is 32 kg/m^2. There is nothing else relevant in her history and on examination.
108. A 22-year-old wishes to go on an effective contraceptive. She is epileptic on lamotrigine which controls her fits very well. Her BMI is normal and her periods are regular.
109. A 34-year-old who has had three children [delivered by cesarean section (CS) as she has a uterine abnormality] wishes to have an effective form of contraception. She says that she does not want more children. She is allergic to metals and also has hypertension for which she is receiving methyldopa. Her sister suffered from a deep vein thrombosis (DVT) while on the combined contraceptive pill 3 years ago.

PRINCIPLES OF SURGERY IN GYNECOLOGY

Option list for questions 110–113

A	Burch colposuspension	G	Myomectomy
B	Cystoscopy	H	Posterior repair
C	Diagnostic laparoscopy	I	Sacrocolpopexy
D	Hysterectomy	J	Sacrospinous fixation
E	Hysteroscopy	K	Surgical evacuation of products of the uterus
F	LLETZ	L	TVT

Instructions: The following are descriptions of surgical procedures to treat various gynecological problems. For each procedure, select from the list of options above the most appropriate term that describes the procedure. Each option may be chosen once, more than once, or not at all.

110. A 34-year-old with heavy and regular menses had an enlarged irregular uterus that measured about 24 weeks of pregnancy size. An ultrasound scan confirmed the presence of multiple masses and she has undergone surgery to ensure that her periods are not heavy and she would also be able to have children.
111. A 50-year-old who had a vaginal hysterectomy 5 years now presents with prolapse of the vaginal vault. She does not have any urinary symptoms and is also sexually active. She has undergone an operation

which will ensure that the prolapse is corrected and her vaginal anatomy is maintained.

112. A 26-year-old who had attended with a history of chronic pelvic pain (CPP) that had failed to respond to medical treatment had surgery to help with finding the cause of the pain and in this case also had treatment.
113. A 47-year-old who presented with stress urinary incontinence and was offered physiotherapy but this failed to alleviate her symptoms. She attended for a day-case procedure to correct the incontinence.

Option list for questions 114–116

A	Inferior epigastric artery	F	Spiral artery
B	Left ovarian vein	G	Uterine artery
C	Ovarian artery	H	Vaginal artery
D	Pudendal artery	I	
E	Right ovarian vein	J	

Instructions: For each of these anatomical descriptions identify the single structure above that represents it. Each option may be chosen once, more than once, or not at all.

114. Drains the ovary directly into the inferior vena cava.
115. Anastomosis with the ovarian artery under the fallopian tube in the mesosalpinx.
116. Most likely to be damaged by the lateral port at laparoscopy.

Part A: Answer and Explanations

1. **(A) Anterior division of the internal iliac.** The main blood supply to the uterus is the uterine artery which is branch of the anterior division of the internal iliac artery. This enters the uterus laterally at the level of the internal os and turns upward to anastomose with the ovarian artery and downward to anastomose with the vaginal artery—both (ovarian and vaginal) of these also supply blood to the uterus.
2. **(C) Left ovarian vein.** The right ovary is drained by a vein which empties into the inferior vena cava while the left ovarian drain empties into the renal vein.
3. **(I) Transverse cervical or cardinal ligament.** The pelvic supporting structures are the muscles of which the levator ani is the main one and the ligaments of which the transverse cervical (cardinal) ligament is the main one. The round ligament maintains the uterus in its anteverted position.
4. **(J) Transabdominal ultrasound scan.** This patient has a suspected abdominal mass which is likely to be a hematocolpos from retained menstruation. A transabdominal ultrasound scan will confirm the diagnosis. As she is likely to be virgo intacta (virgin), a transvaginal ultrasound scan or bimanual examination would be inappropriate. While an MRI can also be useful, it is more costly and takes time to arrange.
5. **(B) Cusco's speculum and endocervical and urethral swabs.** This patient most likely has a sexually transmitted infection (STI) and swabs should be obtained from the cervix and urethra. It is also possible to obtain low vaginal swabs as long as these are for polymerase chain reaction (PCR) test for the various organisms causing STI.
6. **(I) Sims speculum.** This patient presents with symptoms of genital prolapse and should be examined with a Sim's speculum in the left lateral position.
7. **(H) Turner mosaic.** The clinical features are consistent with those of Turner syndrome. The presence of two karyotypes is diagnostic of mosaicism.
8. **(A) Androgen insensitivity syndrome (AIS).** Androgen insensitivity syndrome is characterized by absent female internal genitalia but normal external genitalia. It results from resistance of the androgen receptor or its mediators to binding to testosterone and dihydrotestosterone. Bilateral hernias and scant pubic hair with a short blind-ending vagina are characteristic findings on examination.

9. **(B) Congenital adrenal hyperplasia (CAH).** There are three main type of CAH–21-hydroxylase deficiency, 11β-hydroxylase deficiency, and 3β-hydroxysteroid dehydrogenase deficiency. 21-hydroxylase deficiency is the most common and typically presents at birth with ambiguous external genitalia (hypertrophic clitoris appearing like a phallus, rugged labia majora appearing like scrotum.
10. **(A) Complete miscarriage.** A history of passage of blood clots and liver-like tissue with lower abdominal pains and clinical findings of settled bleeding, closed cervical os, and a suspected normal size uterus are all diagnostic of a complete miscarriage. The urine pregnancy test is still positive as there is still human chorionic gonadotropin (hCG) in the circulation.
11. **(B) Complete molar pregnancy.** The diagnosis of a complete molar pregnancy is supported by the history of excessive vomiting, slight vaginal bleeding, and a uterus that is much larger than dates and with no obvious fetal parts on palpation. The diagnosis will be confirmed by an ultrasound scan showing a snow-storm appearance in the uterine contents.
12. **(E) Inevitable miscarriage.** An inevitable miscarriage is one in which there is a pregnancy in the uterus of a patient presenting with vaginal bleeding, with or without pains and an opened cervical os. The presence of a viable intrauterine pregnancy does not change the diagnosis as the opened os is the diagnostic feature.
13. **(A) Evacuation—surgical.** This patient has an inevitable miscarriage and the management options are: (1) expectant, (2) medical, and (3) surgical—evacuation. The last option is most suitable as she is continuing to bleed and is therefore more likely to become quickly unstable. Furthermore, she is already mildly tachycardic suggesting an already significant blood loss. Expectant or medical management options and reserved for those who are not actively bleeding and are clinically stable.
14. **(D) Methotrexate.** There are three options for managing ectopic pregnancies and these include: (1) expectant management, (2) medical management with methotrexate, and (3) surgical management. Expectant management is offered to those who are stable with quantified hCG of <1,000 IU and an adnexal mass of <35 mm in diameter without a fetal heartbeat. Where the hCG is <1,500 and the patient is stable with an ectopic <35 mm, medical management is preferred (as in this patient) and surgery is reserved for unstable patients, those with high hCG or adnexal masses >35 mm or with fetal heartbeat.
15. **(B) Expectant management.** The options for this patient are either expectant, medical, or surgery. As she is stable and wishes the least invasive treatment, expectant management would be the best option.

She is allowing nature to take its course and this is likely to be successful in up to 80% of cases within 7–14 days.

16. **(F) Serum β-hCG.** This patient has a pregnancy of unknown location which may progress to one of three possibilities—(1) viable and continuing intrauterine pregnancy, (2) an ectopic pregnancy, or (3) failed pregnancy. Quantifying β-hCG will help as if the values are above a threshold for an intrauterine gestational sac, it would most, likely be an ectopic pregnancy. If the values are below the threshold then a repeat after 48 hours would be recommended.
17. **(H) Transvaginal ultrasound scan.** The differential diagnoses in this patient are a viable intrauterine pregnancy or an ectopic pregnancy. At a β-hCG of 3,000 IU, it should be possible to see an intrauterine pregnancy and if this is absent, the diagnosis is most likely that of an ectopic pregnancy. A transabdominal ultrasound will be an option but it would not be as sensitive as a transvaginal sonography (TVS).
18. **(G) Speculum examination.** She has suffered from a vasovagal shock from dilatation of the cervix with products being stuck in the cervix. A speculum examination and removal of the products from the cervix will be followed very quickly by recovery of BP and return of pulse to normal.
19. **(F) Hypothyroidism.** Hypothyroidism is a cause of precious puberty and typically the patients are obese or overweight and complains of poor heat control. A differential diagnosis is Cushing syndrome but patients with this syndrome have a moon-face appearance and hirsutism.
20. **(I) Estrogen-producing ovarian tumor.** The diagnosis here is isolated precious puberty and most likely secondary to estrogen-producing tumors as the development is confined to the breast with no pubic and axillar hair development.
21. **(C) Constitutional.** Precocious puberty is defined as that occurring before the age of 8 years. In females the most common cause is constitutional. She presents with central precocity and no abnormal symptoms. The most likely cause is therefore constitutional.
22. **(A) Adenomyosis.** The clinical presentation—heavy regular periods with dyspareunia and a uniformly enlarged uterus which is not firm excludes uterine fibroids and supports the diagnosis of adenomyosis.
23. **(H) Ovulatory disorder such as in PCOS.** The most likely diagnosis in this patient is PCOS. In these patients, there is high circulating estrogen which causes prolonged overstimulation of the endometrium such that when periods occur they are heavy.
24. **(C) Hysterectomy.** The patient has completed her family, has very large uterine fibroids and has had to be transfused twice because of the heavy menstrual bleeding. A hysterectomy would be the best

treatment for her. Her tubes should also be removed at the same procedure.

25. **(D) Levonorgestrel intrauterine system (IUS) (Mirena®).** The treatment of choice for heavy menstrual bleeding is the levonorgestrel IUS (Mirena®). This is more so in women who have had children and may require this as a form of contraception.
26. **(E) Intrauterine adhesions or Asherman syndrome.** The presentation is typical of Asherman syndrome—surgical evacuation followed by hypomenorrhea and then infertility.
27. **(I) Tubal disease (from infections).** The history of right hypochondrial and lower abdominal pain is suggestive of *chlamydia trachomatis* infection. This is the most common cause of tubal disease infertility. A significant number of those who have had this infection are asymptomatic.
28. **(C) Congenital absence of the vas.** Congenital absence of the vas presents with azoospermia with normal FSH. The only other causes of azoospermia will include radiotherapy, trauma, and genetics—none of which is present in this man.
29. **(F) Serum prolactin.** Headaches and a discharge from the breast suggest a possible intracranial pathology possibly a prolactinoma, hence measurement of serum prolactin would be most appropriate.
30. **(C) Hysterosalpingography (HSG)—tubal patency test.** With an ovulatory biochemistry and a normal semen, the patency of the tubes has to be assessed. The options are diagnostic laparoscopy and dye test or HSG. As she has no symptoms, it is easier to perform an HSG rather than a laparoscopy and dye test.
31. **(E) Semen analysis.** In the investigation of couples with infertility, once the woman has been shown to be ovulating, before further tests are performed a semen analysis should be available and only when this is normal should further tests like tubal patency tests be performed.
32. **(C) Cervical ectropion.** This is a typical presentation of cervical ectropion—intermenstrual and postcoital bleeding and copious vaginal discharge which is watery and worse midcycle. The red cervix is from replacement of the ectocervical squamous epithelium with columnar epithelium of the endocervix.
33. **(B) Asherman syndrome.** Intrauterine adhesions (Asherman syndrome) commonly result from overzealous curettage of the uterus, especially at surgical evacuations. It can also result from myomectomy where the endometrium is breached. Presentation is typically with scanty periods, infertility, or recurrent early miscarriages. Occasionally these can present as preterm labor and placenta accreta.

34. **(A) Adenomyosis.** The history of painful periods starting a few days before the periods and lasting for a few days after suggests either endometriosis of adenomyosis. With endometriosis, the uterus is not usually enlarged unless there is coexisting pathology.
35. **(F) Endometriosis.** Symptoms of endometriosis include painful periods which tend to start a day or 2 before menstruation, reach a crescendo a few days into the period and gradually get better after periods have finished. Findings of examination are variable including nothing, induration of the utero-sacral ligaments, adnexal masses, retroverted fixed or minimally mobile uterus and adnexal masses or tenderness.
36. **(K) Uterine fibroids.** Heavy periods associated with the passage of clots can cause clot dysmenorrhea. The symptoms typically occur when periods are heaviest (usually on days 1–3) as in this patient. The presence of an irregularly firm and enlarged uterus with no adnexal masses or tenderness support the diagnosis.
37. **(J) Primary dysmenorrhea.** Primary dysmenorrhea is painful menstruation with onset at puberty. The pain is typically spasmodic and gets better after the first 2/3 days as in this patient. Her superficial dyspareunia is not related to the dysmenorrhea, especially that lubricants improve the pain.
38. **(D) GnRH antagonist/estradiol/norethindrone.** This patient has endometriosis, and the gold standard treatment is either a GnRH agonists or antagonist. Currently the treatment that has the least side-effects if GnRH antagonist combined with estradiol and norethindrone. As she has tried oral hormonal preparations without success, the only options here are the GnRH agonist or antagonists, Mirena and surgery.
39. **(J) Ovarian cystectomy.** Treatment options in this patient include the medical options of progestogens, GnRH agonist and surgery. Surgery offers the best option of ameliorating her symptoms especially that the cyst measures >5 cm.
40. **(A) Combined hormonal contraception.** The diagnosis in this young girl is primary dysmenorrhea. The treatment options are NSAIDs and combined contraceptives. Although she is not sexually active and there is no information on whether NSAIDs have been tried before the option for her is combined hormonal contraception. NSAIDS maybe considered as first option though.
41. **(G) Granulosa cell tumor.** This girl has features of estrogenization—development of breasts to Tanner stage 3, and vaginal bleeding. Only an estrogen producing ovarian tumor will cause these symptoms. The presence of an ovarian cyst is therefore suggestive of a granulosa cell tumor which can present with precocious puberty or postmenopausal bleeding.

42. **(B) Dermoid ovarian cyst.** Dermoid cysts are benign (matured) teratomas that originate from the embryonal cells hence can contain a variety of tissues including bones, neural and endocrine tissue, skin, teeth and hair. They are also more likely to undergo torsion as they tend to be heavy as was the case in this patient.
43. **(E) Functional ovarian (follicular) cyst.** The classical appearance of a simple functional ovarian cyst is one with thin smooth walls and an echo-free fluid within the cyst. The differential diagnosis includes a serous cystadenoma; however, her age and the symptoms are in keeping with a functional ovarian cyst.
44. **(C) *Chlamydia trachomatis.*** The picture is consistent with chlamydia infection. Although most are asymptomatic, those with symptoms present with upper and lower abdominal pain and dysuria. A pelvic examination may demonstrate tenderness in the lower abdomen and cervical motion tenderness reflects inflammation of the pelvis.
45. **(E) Herpes simplex.** The presence of painful blisters on the vulva is diagnostic of herpes simplex infection. Acute urinary retention is an uncommon presentation and is often related to pain.
46. **(F) Nucleic acid amplification (NAAT).** Nucleic acid amplification test—a PCR test will allow for quick diagnosis of STIs including *Chlamydia trachomatis* and *Neisseria gonorrhoeae.* It does not however provide antibiotic sensitivity.
47. **(G) Nontreponemal test.** Screening for HIV and syphilis are routine investigations offered to women when they book for antenatal care. As this woman recently had a test for HIV she does not require a fourth-generation test (which is for HIV); however, she requires a nontreponemal test [either the rapid plasma reagin or venereal disease research laboratory (VDRL) test]. If this is positive, then a Treponema Pallidum Hemagglutination Assay (TPHA) test would be required.
48. **(D) Fluid for viral PCR.** The most likely diagnosis in this patient is herpes simplex and the diagnosis can be confirmed quickly by viral PCR. Dark-field microscopy is another diagnostic approach, but this does not generate results quickly.
49. **(C) Benzathine penicillin.** The diagnosis in this patient is syphilis and the treatment of choice is benzathine penicillin. If she is allergic to this then doxycycline or ceftriaxone would be other options.
50. **(A) Aciclovir.** The treatment of choice for those presenting with *Herpes simplex virus* (HSV) is acyclovir. This reduces the viral load and symptoms. This can be given orally.
51. **(D) Ceftriaxone.** The treatment of *N. gonorrhoeae* is either a single dose of Ceftriaxone or a combination of ciprofloxacin and penicillin. A single dose treatment is associated with a better outcome.

52. **(I) Rescreen in 12 months.** Current screening is based on testing for HR-HPV. If this is negative, the patients will be referred for routine recall (3 or 5 years) depending on her age. If HR-HPV is positive then the patient will have reflex cytology. Following a negative cytology, screening is repeated after 12 months and if the cytology is other than normal then referral to colposcopy is recommended. If at colposcopy treatment is offered follow-up is at 6 months with HPV testing whereas if no treatment is offered, follow-up is after 12 months
53. **(B) Colposcopy.** Same explanation as for question 51.
54. **(H) Rescreen after 6 months.** Same explanation as for question 51.
55. **(A) Back to routine recall screening (3–5 years).** Same explanation as for question 51.
56. **(F) Lichen sclerosus.** This is an autoimmune condition which typically affects prepubertal or postmenopausal women. It presents with vulva itching, soreness, and painful sexual intercourse. The appearance of the vulva is typically pale/whitish, atrophic with fusion of the labia minor as in this patient. Treatment is with topical corticosteroids.
57. **(B) Dermatitis (vulva eczema).** Eczematous lesions of the vulva could be secondary to atopy (as in patients with allergy conditions such as hay fever or asthma) or secondary to irritants from chemicals or various agents. In this patient, the symptoms date back to the use of specific cream and exposure to possible irritants.
58. **(I) Vulvodynia.** This is a form of discomfort vulva in which the patient presents with a burning sensation, especially on touching in the absence of pathology. It can either be localized or generalized. Sexual intercourse is usually very painful (superficial dyspareunia) and in most cases the patients avoid it all together. The diagnosis is based on a positive provocative test. Treatment is with local anesthetic agents or tricyclic antidepressants.
59. **(A) Bacterial vaginosis.** Bacterial vaginosis presents with an offensive discharge which sticks to the vagina and sometimes has a fishy smell. The pH of the vagina is >4.5 and a diagnostic feature on microscopy is the present of clue cells.
60. **(G) *Trichomonas vaginalis.*** This protozoal infection presents with a scanty to profuse discharge which is offensive and appears frothy and greenish to yellowish. Itching and soreness may coexist with the discharge. The vaginal pH is >4.5 and a strawberry cervix is pathognomonic.
61. **(H) *Vulvovaginal candidiasis.*** A history of type II diabetes, recurrent nonoffensive whitish discharge associated with itching and the cottage cheese appearance of the vagina are diagnostic of vulvovaginal candidiasis. The pH of the vagina in these cases is usually <4.5.

62. **(C) Cone biopsy.** For stage 1A1 disease with invasion <3 mm, the treatment of choice is cone biopsy. In this patient who desires fertility preservation, this is the most appropriate treatment as it will not significantly affect fertility.
63. **(F) Radical hysterectomy (Wertheim's hysterectomy).** The treatment of choice for stage IB-II is Wertheim's or radical hysterectomy. This procedure involves removal of the uterus, the parametrium, upper cuff of the vaginal and pelvic lymph nodes with preservation of the ovaries.
64. **(D) External radiotherapy and brachytherapy (intracavitary).** For advanced cervical disease the treatment is usually by radiotherapy (external beam and internal or intracavitary radiation) and/or combined with chemotherapy (chemoradiotherapy).
65. **(F) Stage IIA1.** Stage II carcinoma involves the cervix and spread to the upper two-thirds of the vagina only (IIA) or parametrium but not up to the pelvic side wall (IIB). Where stromal invasion is <4 cm it is IIA1 and if >4 cm it is IIA2.
66. **(J) Stage IIIB.** Stage III cancer involves the lower vagina (IIIA) or spread to the side wall (IIIB). Where lymph nodes are involved it is stage IIIC.
67. **(A) Stage 1A1.** Cervical cancer that is confined to the cervix and diagnosed only on microscopy is microscopic and where stromal invasion is <3 mm it is staged as 1A1 and if the stromal invasion is 3–5 mm it is stage 1A2.
68. **(D) Endometrial hyperplasia without atypia.** Treatment of endometrial hyperplasia is with progestogens–oral for that without hyperplasia and local (intrauterine) if surgery is declined in those with hyperplasia and atypia.
69. **(C) Endometrial hyperplasia with atypia.** This patient most likely was offered a hysterectomy and BSO for hyperplasia with atypia and as she desires fertility sparing treatment, the best option would be a locally acting progestogen such as the levonorgestrel IUS (Mirena®).
70. **(H) Well-differentiated adenocarcinoma.** This is the most common type of endometrial cancer and treated with hysterectomy and BSO.
71. **(A) Stage 1A.** Stage 1 endometrial carcinoma is cancer confined to the uterus. This is further classified into 1A if <50% of the myometrium is invaded and 1B if >50% of the myometrium is invaded by the cancer. Lymphovascular invasion does no influence this staging.
72. **(C) Stage II.** Cancer of the endometrium that has spread to the cervical stroma is stage II disease as long as it does not extend beyond the uterus.
73. **(H) Stage IVA.** Stage IV disease involves spread to the bladder/rectum but confined to the pelvis (Stage IVA) or intra-abdominal, distant, or inguinal nodes metastasis (IVB).

74. **(D) Granulosa cell tumor.** This is an estrogen producing tumor and the raised inhibin level is diagnostic of a granulosa cell tumor. This can present with precocious puberty in the young age group, irregular period during the reproductive years, and postmenopausal bleeding as in this patient.
75. **(G) Serous cystadenocarcinoma.** Serous cystadenocarcinoma is the most common surface epithelial tumor and one with the highest familial tendency. Hereditary cancers are more likely to be adenocarcinomas that present later in life.
76. **(H) Sertoli–Leydig tumor.** She presents with features of androgenization (hirsutism deepening of her voice and amenorrhea). The rapid onset of these symptoms and the findings on clinical and imaging examination point to an androgen producing tumor.
77. **(A) Stage 1A.** Stage 1 ovarian cancer is confined to one (1A) or both ovaries (1B) without malignant cells in ascitic or peritoneal washings or (1C) if one or both ovaries and there are malignant cells in ascitic fluid or peritoneal washings or the cyst is ruptured during surgery.
78. **(C) Stage 1C1.** Stage 1 ovarian cancer is confined to one (1A) or both ovaries (1B) without malignant cells in ascitic or peritoneal washings or (1C) if one or both ovaries and there are malignant cells in ascitic fluid or peritoneal washings or the cyst is ruptured during surgery. When it is ruptured during surgery it is stage 1C1.
79. **(J) Stage IIIB.** Stage 1 ovarian cancer is confined to one or both ovaries, stage II confined to the ovaries and pelvic extension or peritoneal cancer (limited to the pelvis), stage III cancer involves extra-pelvic but intra-abdominal spread, which could be IIIA with retroperitoneal node involvement (on cytology or histology), IIIB with macroscopic intraperitoneal spread and stage IV with distance metastasis excluding peritoneal metastasis.
80. **(A) Stage Ia.** Stage I vulva cancer is that which is confined to the vulva or perineum with invasion of <1 mm and negative nodes. This is further divided into Ia if the lesion is <2 cm and Ib if it is >2 cm.
81. **(C) Stage II.** Stage II vulva cancer is cancer which has spread to involve adjacent structures but confirmed to one-third of the lower urethra or one-third of the lower vaginal or anus but with negative nodes.
82. **(K) Stage IVb.** Stage III vulva cancer is cancer with involvement of lymph nodes but with no distant metastases. In stage IV disease there is lymph node involvement as well as distant metastasis. Spread to adjacent structures only is stage IV(i) but that which is beyond adjacent structures is stage IVb.

83. **(A) Biopsy for histology.** The most important investigation to perform at this stage is a biopsy to confirm the diagnosis. Once this has been done, then other investigations that will help plan and manage her would be required. These will include a FBC, liver function test (LFT), chest X-ray, and MRI to help stage the cancer.
84. **(G) MRI of the pelvis and abdomen.** Having made a histological diagnosis, the next step must be staging the cancer. This is best achieved through and MRI of the pelvis and abdomen. This will identify spread beyond the vaginal wall, lymph node involvement and any metastases to the liver. Although PET scans are better at defining lymph node spread, they are not as good as MRI in defining local spread.
85. **(H) Positron emission tomography (PET) scan.** Recurrence of disease is best monitored with PET scans while pretreatment spread is best defined with MRI.
86. **(J) Radical wide excision and ipsilateral lymph node dissection.** The diagnosis has already been made and she has had various investigations to defined local spread. The lesion is >2 cm from the midline and as there are no lymph nodes, it would be considered early-stage disease. Treatment for this is surgery—radical wide excision with ipsilateral groin node dissection.
87. **(A) Adjuvant radiotherapy.** Following surgery, adjuvant radiotherapy is indicated if the microscopic surgery free margin is <8 mm or there are two or more lymph nodes involved. In this patient, the margin is only 5 mm and there are three nodes hence she would benefit from adjuvant radiotherapy.
88. **(K) Radiotherapy.** The cornerstone for treatment of carcinoma of the vagina is radiotherapy. This is usually in the form of combined external beam radiation therapy (EBRT) and intracavitary radiotherapy (ICRT) or brachytherapy. If the cancer is limited to stage I, the treatment is radical hysterectomy and vaginectomy and pelvic lymphadenectomy.
89. **(A) Stage Ia.** Stage I carcinoma of the vulva is one where the cancer is limited to the vagina. It is Ia if the lesion is <2 cm and Ib if it is >2 cm.
90. **(E) Stage III.** Stage III vaginal cancer refers to cancer that is of any size that is growing into the pelvic wall and/or growing into the lower one-thirds of the vagina and has/or blocked the flow of urine (hydronephrosis) that may be causing kidney problems. The nearby nodes are involved but not distant nodes.
91. **(G) Moisturizers.** The woman's symptoms are mainly local and these should be managed initially with moisturizers. In most cases this would be adequate but if it fails, she could be offered topical estrogen preparations.
92. **(B) Combined estrogen and progestogen.** This patient has significant symptoms including loss of libido. Nonhormonal preparations

have been tried unsuccessfully hence the only options are estrogen preparations. Because she has not had a hysterectomy, unopposed estrogen would not be a good option for her. Her systemic symptoms also require more than a topical application.

93. **(F) Lifestyle and dietary modification.** This patient has predominantly vasomotor symptoms. She has comorbidities of diabetes and hypertension and by virtue of her high BMI is at an increased risk of endometrial cancer. Unopposed systemic estrogens are therefore not suitable unless all options have been exhausted. The first and best approach will be lifestyle and dietary modifications including weight management, exercises, and reducing warm clothing.
94. **(H) Urinalysis.** Any patient presenting with urinary incontinence, especially those with symptoms suggestive of overactive bladder should have a urinalysis first. This is because symptoms of urinary tract infection (UTI) may mimic those of an overactive bladder and furthermore urodynamics would be inadvisable until the infection has been treated.
95. **(E) 3-day voiding diary.** This is an important investigation as it allows the establishment of a baseline of the severity of symptoms, details of fluid intake, and severity of symptoms.
96. **(F) Ultrasound scan of the bladder, kidneys, and ureters.** The most likely reason for this patient's symptoms is overflow incontinence. This is common following delivery especially in patients who have had an epidural. If she has not been investigated for infections, urinalysis would be most appropriate. However, it is important to establish what the bladder volume is before and after she has voided.
97. **(C) Mixed urinary incontinence.** The history is suggestive of mixed incontinence—stress incontinence was the predominant symptom at the outset but there is superimposed on this, symptoms of an overactive bladder—urgency, urge incontinence, and frequency of micturition. In such patients, it is important to exclude a UTI as this may mimic the symptoms of an overactive bladder.
98. **(G) Urodynamic stress incontinence.** She presents with the classical features of urodynamic stress incontinence. These patients typically have a weakness of the neck of the bladder and become incontinent when the intra-abdominal pressure is raised as with coughing, sneezing, or lifting (as with this patient). Urinary frequency is normal and there is no nocturia. A 3-day voiding diary will show normal voiding volumes and frequency.
99. **(E) Overactive bladder.** Detrusor overactivity presents with urinary frequency, urgency, urge incontinence, and nocturia. A frequency and voiding diary (3-day voiding diary) will demonstrate an increased voiding frequency (more than eight times per day) and nocturia of

more than one to two/night. In most of these patients, the volume of urine passed tends to be small.

100. **(G) Pelvic floor exercises.** This is the first treatment option for any patient presenting with urinary incontinence irrespective of the type of incontinence.
101. **(C) Bladder retraining.** Following the diagnosis of an overactive bladder the patient should be offered conservative management in the form of counseling on fluid intake (reduction in caffeine drinks), pelvic floor exercises, and most importantly bladder retraining.
102. **(F) Duloxetine.** The first treatment for any urinary incontinence is conservative consisting of pelvic floor exercises, reduction in weight and caffeine intake, and bladder retraining. If this fails, then medical treatment with drugs such as duloxetine would be the next option.
103. **(D) Posterior repair.** This patient has a symptomatic rectocele with a normal anatomically situated uterus. A repair of the rectocele is all that would be required in this case. A pessary (ring) may be tried but it is not the most appropriate approach to managing her symptoms.
104. **(A) Anterior repair.** This patient has a prolapse of the anterior compartment (the lower part) which is causing urinary frequency and incomplete emptying of the bladder. The treatment options include surgery (anterior repair) and pessary support. However, the pessary would not be ideal for her but could be used as the first option.
105. **(C) Colpocleisis.** This patient has a stage IV prolapse or procidentia. Surgery is the only treatment option as no conservative approach would be suitable. However, she is frail and unsuitable for any prolonged surgery and one that would also require prolonged postoperative recovery. A colpocleisis would be a quick procedure that would correct the prolapse.
106. **(C) Combined hormonal contraceptive ring.** This patient has painful periods the pattern of which is suggestive of endometriosis. The combined hormonal contraception will be ideal and whether this is taken orally, transdermally or vaginally will be depend on her. As she is not keen on regular medication, an ideal option will be the monthly ring.
107. **(B) Combined contraceptive pill.** This patient has PCOS and wishes contraception. The combined hormonal contraception is effective in treating hirsutism, acne, as well as regularizing her periods. This can be taken orally, transdermally, or vaginally. However, for her symptoms, the best option is oral.
108. **(K) Subdermal implant (Nexplanon).** In this patient, a contraceptive that would not be affected by her antiepileptic is ideal. Additionally, a contraceptive that does not require frequent administration preferable. The subdermal implant is the most effective contraceptive and one

that is not affected by the antiepileptic medication as well as having no effect on the epilepsy.

109. **(I) Sterilization—female.** This woman has completed her family. Her uterine abnormality makes the IUDs unsuitable. Her history is a relative contraindication to hormonal contraceptives especially the combined form. As she is allergic to metals, the copper IUD is unsuitable. The best option for her is therefore sterilization.
110. **(G) Myomectomy.** An enlarged uterus which is irregular on palpation is most likely secondary to fibroids. These will cause heavy and regular periods. Myomectomy is removal of the fibroids which will deal with the heavy periods and also preserve the uterus and thus her fertility.
111. **(I) Sacrocolpopexy.** Vault prolapse is treated by either sacrospinous fixation or sacrocolpopexy. The former is a vagina approach with a shorter hospital stay but the vagina is angled and therefore sexual intercourse may be difficult. Sacrocolpopexy is done by laparotomy or laparoscopically and is associated with maintenance of the vaginal anatomy but morbidity is greater after surgery.
112. **(C) Diagnostic laparoscopy.** In this patient the procedure is a diagnostic laparoscopy as this allows for diagnosis and where possible treatment. The most likely finding would have been endometriosis which might have been excised or diathermied.
113. **(L) TVT.** Women with stress urinary incontinence should be offered physiotherapy first. When this fails then sling procedures such as TVTs or colposuspension should be offered. In the first instance, the TVTs (tension-free vaginal tapes or transobturator tapes) should be used and if these fail then Burch colposuspension should be considered.
114. **(E) Right ovarian vein.** The ovarian veins drain into different structure—the left drains into the renal vein while the right drains into the inferior vena cava.
115. **(G) Uterine artery.** The uterine artery enters the uterus at the level of the internal cervical os and branches upward giving off the spiral artery which penetrates to supply the myometrium. It then continues upward to anastomose with the ovarian artery in the mesosalpinx.
116. **(A) Inferior epigastric artery.** The epigastric arteries are most likely to be damaged by lateral ports at laparoscopy because of their anatomical location.

Part B: Single Best Answer Questions

BASIC EMBRYOLOGY

1. After what gestational age do the gonads become differentiated?

A. 6 weeks
B. 7 weeks
C. 8 weeks
D. 9 weeks
E. 10 weeks

2. At what gestational age is the number of primordial follicles maximum in females?

A. 10 weeks
B. 15 weeks
C. 20 weeks
D. 28 weeks
E. 36 weeks

3. Which congenital abnormality of the genital tract is likely to present with primary cyclical lower abdominal pain and amenorrhea?

A. Arcuate uterus
B. Bicornuate uterus
C. Imperforate hymen
D. Unicornuate uterus
E. Uterine didelphys

BASIC ANATOMY AND PHYSIOLOGY OF REPRODUCTION

4. Which structures lie anterior to the uterus during the reproductive years?

A. Bladder
B. Bladder and bowel
C. Bladder, bowel, and fascia
D. Bladder, bowel, and ovary
E. Bladder, bowel, and ureters

5. The fallopian tube is divided into several parts. Which part of the tube is intramuscular?

A. Ampullary portion
B. Fimbrial portion
C. Interstitial portion
D. Isthmus
E. Tubal ostium

6. What happens to the ovaries after menopause?

A. The shrink in size
B. The change their location to the pelvic brim
C. They contain few follicles
D. Their surface becomes smooth and shiny
E. They change shape from almond to round

GYNECOLOGY HISTORY AND PHYSICAL EXAMINATION

7. A thorough gynecological examination should start with inspection. Which of the following pairs are part of the inspection process?

A. Sims speculum examination and the patient in the dorsal position
B. Cusco's (bivalve) speculum and the patient in the lateral position
C. Exposure of the chest and examination of the apex of the heart
D. Dorsal position and inspection of the labia
E. Dorsal position and transabdominal ultrasound scan

8. A patient comes to the clinic with a vaginal discharge and lower abdominal pains. The plan is to take a swab for culture and sensitivity. What is the best time to take the swab in the course of examining this patient?

A. After a bimanual examination to determine if there is cervical motion tenderness
B. After a digital check that the vaginal is able to accommodate the speculum
C. After inserting a speculum lubricated with an antiseptic
D. After inserting a speculum lubricated with gel or water
E. When the vulva is being inspected

PUBERTY AND PUBERTAL DISORDERS

9. At what age does normal puberty start in girls?

A. 6–7 years
B. 7–8 years
C. 8–9 years
D. 9–10 years
E. 10–11 years

10. A 7-year-old is brought by her mother with complaints of breasts development of 3 months duration. What is the most likely cause of this if she does not have any other features of pubertal development?

A. Constitutional
B. Part of normal pubertal development
C. Adrenal disorder
D. Ovarian estrogen producing tumor
E. Iatrogenic (from drugs)

11. A 16-year-old attends with primary amenorrhea and normal secondary sexual characteristics. She does not have any lower abdominal pains. When examined she has well developed secondary sex characteristics (normal height, breasts, and pubic hair) and no palpable abdominal masses. What is the most likely cause of the amenorrhea?

A. Atresia of the lower genital tract
B. Chromosome abnormality
C. Congenital adrenal hyperplasia
D. Gonadal dysgenesis
E. Mullerian agenesis

12. What is the most important investigation to perform on a newborn baby with external ambiguous genitalia?

A. Blood glucose
B. Buccal smear for bar body
C. Electrolyte and urea
D. Ultrasound of the abdomen and pelvis
E. Karyotype from peripheral lymphocytes

13. What is the karyotype of a 13-year-old who is short-statured, has wide carrying angles of the upper limbs and a coarctation of the aorta?

A. 45XO
B. 46XX
C. 46XX+13
D. 26XX+18
E. 46XX+21

MENSTRUATION PHYSIOLOGY AND DISORDERS OF MENSTRUATION

14. What best describe the hormonal changes in the hypothalamic-ovarian axis that result in ovulation?

A. High progesterone and high estradiol leading to preovulatory LH surge
B. Increase in progesterone followed by a rise in LH
C. Low estradiol and progesterone levels leading to preovulatory LH and FSH surge
D. Low progesterone and high estradiol leading to a preovulatory surge in FSH and LH
E. Low progesterone and high estradiol leading to a preovulatory surge in LH

15. How long prior to ovulation does the LH surge occur?

A. 12–24 hours
B. 12–36 hours
C. 20–36 hours
D. 24–36 hours
E. 24–48 hours

16. What is responsible for the recruitment of follicles at the beginning of the next menstrual cycle?

A. Low estradiol levels
B. Low estradiol and inhibin levels
C. Low estradiol and progesterone
D. Low progesterone, inhibin levels
E. Low progesterone, inhibin, and estradiol levels

EARLY PREGNANCY COMPLICATIONS

17. A 24-year-old is seen in the emergency at 8 weeks amenorrhea with mild vaginal bleeding and cramps. This is her first pregnancy. She had a pregnancy test at home which was positive. She is examined and there is some blood in the vagina and the cervical os is closed. On bimanual examination the uterus is about 8 weeks in size. What is the most likely diagnosis?

A. Complete miscarriage
B. Incomplete miscarriage
C. Inevitable miscarriage
D. Missed miscarriage
E. Threatened miscarriage

18. What is the most common cause of recurrent miscarriages?

A. Antiphospholipid syndrome
B. Chromosomal abnormalities
C. Medical disorders in the woman
D. Unexplained
E. Uterine abnormalities

19. A 30-year-old is seen in the EPAU at 8 weeks amenorrhea with mild cramps and vaginal bleeding. She is examined and found to have a closed cervical os, a bulky uterus, and adnexal tenderness. What would be the next investigation to help make a diagnosis?

A. Quantified serum hCG
B. Quantified urine hCG
C. Transabdominal ultrasound scan
D. Transvaginal ultrasound scan
E. Urine pregnancy test

20. What would be the recommended first management option for a 26-year-old woman with a diagnosis of a missed miscarriage at 10 weeks of pregnancy who is not bleeding and is able to come back for repeated follow-up?

A. Expectant management
B. Manual suction evacuation
C. Medical management with misoprostol and anti-progestogen (mifepristone)
D. Methotrexate
E. Surgical suction evacuation

21. A 19-year-old woman presents with left sided lower abdominal pains and a dirty brown vaginal discharge. Her periods are irregular and the last one was about 6 weeks ago. She does not complain of any other symptoms. On examination, she is tender in the lower abdomen and there is positive cervical motion tenderness on the

left side and the uterus is marginally enlarged. A urine pregnancy test is positive. What is the most likely diagnosis?

A. Complete miscarriage
B. Ectopic pregnancy
C. Missed miscarriage
D. Septic miscarriage
E. Threatened miscarriage

22. When should anti-D be administered to a woman whose blood group is Rhesus (D) negative presenting with an early pregnancy complication?

A. She has a complete miscarriage at 10 weeks of gestation
B. She has a medically managed miscarriage at 10 weeks of gestation
C. She has a surgically managed miscarriage at 10 weeks of gestation
D. She has an ectopic pregnancy that is managed surgically
E. She presents with a threatened miscarriage with a history of passage of blood clots but with settled bleeding at 10 weeks of gestation

23. Which type of gestational trophoblastic disease is of paternal origin only?

A. Complete molar pregnancy
B. Epithelioid trophoblastic tumor
C. Incomplete molar pregnancy
D. Placental site nodule
E. Placental site trophoblastic tumor

24. A 22-year-old woman had an evacuation for a complete molar pregnancy at 10 weeks of gestation. What should she be told about when to get pregnant again?

A. To avoid pregnancy for 6 weeks
B. To avoid pregnancy for 6 months
C. To avoid pregnancy for 6 months from evacuation if hCG returns to normal within 56 days
D. To avoid pregnancy for 12 months from evacuation

25. Which contraception is not recommended for immediate use by a woman who has had a surgical evacuation of a complete molar pregnancy at 12 weeks of gestation?

A. Combined hormonal contraception
B. Progestogen only oral contraception
C. Subdermal progestogen implant
D. Depo-Provera
E. Barrier method of contraception

GASTROINTESTINAL DISORDERS IN PREGNANCY (CONSTIPATION, NAUSEA, AND VOMITING)

26. What would recommend in the first instance for a 30-year-old woman multiparous mother of three who presents with constipation at 30 weeks of gestation?

A. Bulk forming agents
B. Dietary modifications
C. Osmotic laxatives
D. Stimulant laxatives
E. Suppositories

27. When will you diagnosed hyperemesis gravidarum in any patient presenting with nausea and vomiting in early pregnancy?

A. She presents with vomiting that is associated with dehydration
B. She presents with vomiting that is associated with a weight loss of >5%
C. She presents with vomiting that is associated with weight loss of >5%, electrolyte disturbance and dehydration
D. She presents with vomiting, weight loss of at least 10%, and electrolyte imbalance
E. She presents with intractable vomiting associated with weight loss of >10%, electrolyte derangement, and dehydration

28. What will be the initial treatment of choice for a primigravida who presents at 7 weeks with nausea and vomiting? She has lost 2% of her prepregnancy weight and on examination is not dehydrated. Her urea and electrolytes are normal.

A. Intravenous rehydration
B. Oral cyclizine
C. Oral metoclopramide
D. Oral ondansetron
E. Oral rehydration

PUBERTY AND PUBERTAL DISORDERS

29. At what stage of puberty does menstruation start?

A. Stage 1
B. Stage 2
C. Stage 3
D. Stage 4
E. Stage 5

30. What is the most common cause of precocious puberty in females?

A. Adrenal tumors
B. Constitutional
C. Disorders of the central nervous system (congenital or acquired)
D. Medical disorders
E. Tumors of the ovary

31. At what age will you diagnose delayed puberty in a girl who has no secondary sexual characteristics?

A. 12 years
B. 13 years
C. 14 years
D. 15 years
E. 16 years

32. A 16-year-old girl presents with failure of development of secondary sexual characteristics. She is examined and found to be short-statured, with widespread breast and coarctation of the aorta. She has a karyotype as part of investigations. What is the karyotype associated with this phenotype?

A. 45XO
B. 45XO/46XX
C. 46XXX
D. 46, XY DSD
E. 47XX+21

33. An 8-year-old girl attends with her mother complaining that she has been menstruating for the past 6 months. Her two sisters started menstruating at the ages of 12 and 13 years. She gives a history of pubertal development that follows an expected normal pattern. She is examined and found to have normal secondary sexual characteristics and nothing abnormal. What would be treatment recommended for this girl?

A. Antiestrogens
B. Continuous progestogens
C. Cortisol
D. GnRH agonist
E. Reassurance

DISORDERS OF MENSTRUATION OR ABNORMAL UTERINE BLEEDING

34. When will you make a diagnosis of primary amenorrhea in a young girl presenting to the gynecology clinic with her mother?

A. She is aged 12 years and is yet to start menstruating
B. She is aged 13 years and is yet to start menstruating
C. She is aged 14 years and is yet to start menstruating
D. She is aged 15 years and is yet to start menstruating
E. She is aged 16 years and is yet to start menstruating

35. A 16-year-old girl attends complaining that she is yet to start menstruating. All her secondary sexual characteristics developed at the right time. She says that she started experiencing cyclical lower abdominal pain which is getting worse since she was 13 years old. When examined she is found to have a lower abdominal mass palpable just above the symphysis pubis and a bulge which is bluish-red on separating the labia minora. What is the most likely diagnosis?

A. Cervical stenosis with hematocolpos
B. Double uterus with hematocolpos in one horn
C. Hematocolpos in a rudimentary horn of the Müllerian system
D. Imperforate hymen with hematometra and hematocolpos
E. Vaginal agenesis with hematocolpos

36. A patient is seen in the clinic complaining of excessive hair on her face, abdomen and thighs. She is overweight and her periods are irregular. Her mother suffers from excessive hair growth on her face and has to shave regularly. What is the most likely cause of her symptoms?
A. Adrenal tumor
B. Androgen-producing ovarian tumor
C. Cushing syndrome
D. Familiar (constitutional)
E. Polycystic ovary syndrome (PCOS)

37. What treatment should you start with in the management of a patient whose BMI is 28 kg/m^2 with PCOS and whose predominant symptom is hirsutism?
A. Antiandrogen such as cyproterone acetate
B. Bleaching
C. Combined oral contraceptive
D. Laser treatment
E. Mechanical treatment such as shaving

38. What is the most common cause of secondary dysmenorrhea in a 35-year-old woman who has never been pregnant?
A. Adenomyosis
B. Endometriosis
C. Clot dysmenorrhea
D. Fibroids
E. PID

39. A 27-year-old woman presents with cyclical symptoms which include mood swings, depression, anxiety, loss of sleep, and painful breast. What would be the best approach to making a diagnosis of premenstrual syndrome (PMS)?
A. Confirmation that she is ovulating by ultrasound scan
B. Mapping her symptoms to her periods
C. Symptom diary for 3 months
D. Therapeutic trial with combined hormonal contraception
E. Therapeutic trial with selective serotonin reuptake inhibitors (SSRIs)

40. A 30-year-old woman presents to the clinic with heavy menstrual bleeding. She is examined and found to have an abdominal mass which is firm and irregular arising from the pelvis. Her periods are regular but very heavy. Up to 12 months ago, they were normal. What is the most likely cause of her heavy periods?

A. Adenomyosis
B. Congenital uterine malformation
C. Endometriosis
D. Ovarian cysts
E. Uterine fibroids

41. What single important investigation should be performed first on a 30-year-old patient with heavy menstrual bleeding and a mass arising from the pelvis?

A. Complete blood count (CBC)
B. Endometrial biopsy
C. Transabdominal ultrasound can
D. Transvaginal ultrasound scan
E. Urea and electrolytes

42. A postmenopausal woman comes to the clinic complaining of bleeding for the past 1 month. The uterus is normal in size on vaginal examination. What important investigation should be undertaken in this woman?

A. Endometrial biopsy
B. Complete blood count (CBC)
C. An outpatient hysteroscopy
D. Thyroid function test
E. Transabdominal ultrasound scan for endometrial thickness

SUBFERTILITY

43. How long does the sperm survive in the female genital tract after sexual intercourse?

A. 1 day
B. 2 days
C. 3 days
D. 4 days
E. 5 days

44. A couple attended the clinic because they have been trying unsuccessfully for a pregnancy. The man is aged 30 years and the woman 26 years. When will this couple be labeled as suffering from primary infertility?

A. They have been trying for 6 months
B. They have been trying for 9 months
C. They have been trying for 12 months

D. They have been trying for 18 months
E. They have been trying for 24 months

45. What proportion of infertility is caused by a male factor alone?

A. 5%
B. 10%
C. 15%
D. 20%
E. 30%

46. A couple attend for infertility of 18 months duration. The woman has irregular cycles and also complaints of hirsutism and excessive weight gain. The man smokes 20–30 cigarettes per day. The woman has a BMI of 38 kg/m^2. She is found to have anovulatory cycles while the semen analysis on the man is normal. What would be the first approach to managing this couple?

A. Advice the woman to lose weight
B. Aromatase inhibitor
C. Bariatric surgery for the woman
D. Clomiphene citrate induction of ovulation
E. Metformin

BENIGN CONDITIONS OF THE UTERUS

47. What is the most common tumor of the female genital tract?

A. Adenomyosis
B. Dermoid cysts
C. Endometrial cancer
D. Leiomyoma
E. Ovarian cancer

48. Which type of fibroid is most likely to present with irregular vaginal bleeding?

A. Broad-ligament
B. Intramural
C. Pedunculated intrauterine
D. Submucosal
E. Subserous

49. What is the most common complication of fibroids in pregnancy?

A. Fatty degeneration
B. Hyaline degeneration
C. Impaction in the pelvis
D. Cystic degeneration
E. Red degeneration

50. What is the most common symptom of uterine fibroids?

A. Abdominal mass
B. Asymptomatic, i.e., identified incidentally
C. Heavy and regular menstruation
D. Intermenstrual bleeding
E. Painful periods

51. A 37-year-old woman has been diagnosed with multiple uterine fibroids and is being counseled about myomectomy. What particular complication must accept and acknowledge prior to signing the consent form?

A. Hemorrhage
B. Hysterectomy
C. Infections
D. Infertility
E. Injury to viscera

ENDOMETRIOSIS AND CHRONIC PELVIC PAIN

52. Endometriosis is a common gynecological problem in the reproductive age group. Several theories have been proposed for its pathogenesis. Which of these theories explains the location of endometriosis in the pelvis and uterosacral ligaments?

A. Coelomic metaplasia theory of Meyer
B. Genetic theory
C. Immunologic theory
D. Implantation theory of Sampson
E. Lymphatic spread theory
F. Vascular spread theory

53. A 27-year-old woman presents with painful periods and painful sexual intercourse. The pain during intercourse is experienced after penetration. When examined she is found to have a retroverted immobile but normal size uterus, induration of the uterosacral ligaments, and bilateral adnexal tenderness. Endometriosis is suspected. Which investigation is most likely to confirm the diagnosis?

A. Diagnostic laparoscopy
B. Magnetic resonance imaging (MRI) of the abdomen and pelvis
C. Serum CA125
D. Transabdominal ultrasound scan of the pelvis
E. Transvaginal ultrasound scan of the pelvis

54. What is the treatment of choice in a 20-year-old student with a diagnosis of endometriosis associated with heavy periods?

A. Combined hormonal contraception
B. GnRH agonists
C. Progestogen only tablets
D. Surgical ablation or excision
E. The levonorgestrel intrauterine system (Mirena)

55. A young woman has been referred to the Gynecology outpatients with a diagnosis of CPP. What is the definition of CPP?

A. Pain that in the lower abdomen or pelvis of at least 3 months duration
B. Pain that in the lower abdomen or pelvis of at least 6 months duration
C. Pain that in the lower abdomen or pelvis of at least 12 months duration
D. Pain that in the lower abdomen or pelvis of at least 3 months duration that is not exclusively during menstruation
E. Pain that in the lower abdomen or pelvis of at least 6 months duration that is not exclusively during menstruation

BENIGN OVARIAN DISORDERS

56. What is the most common type of benign ovarian cyst in women aged 15–25 years?

A. Dermoid
B. Serous cystadenoma
C. Mucinous cystadenoma
D. Brenner tumors
E. Fibromas

57. A 23-year-old woman is admitted with sudden-onset acute left-sided lower abdominal pain which started 6 hours ago. The pain is intermittent and associated with nausea and vomiting. Her periods are regular and the last one was 7 days ago. She is sexually active and her boyfriend uses the condom. There has been no abnormal vaginal discharge. When examined there is tenderness on the left side with a possible mass felt. What is the most likely cause of the pain?

A. Acute PID
B. Ectopic pregnancy
C. Hemorrhagic corpus luteum cyst
D. Ovarian cyst torsion
E. Ruptured ovarian cyst

58. An ultrasound scan has been performed on a 28-year-old woman who presented with CPP associated with deep dyspareunia. Her periods are regular but painful with the pain lasting for about 1 week from the start of her periods. She is not using any form of contraception. The scan shows a cystic mass measuring 6 × 8 cm with a ground-glass appearance on the left pelvic side wall. Her last menstrual period (LMP) was 2 weeks ago. What is the most likely diagnosis?

A. Dermoid cyst
B. Endometrioma
C. Hemorrhage ovarian cyst
D. Mucinous cystadenoma
E. Serous cystadenoma

59. A 24-year-old woman presents with lower abdominal pain of 2 days duration. She is sexually active and her LMP was 3 weeks ago. Her periods are irregular. She also says that she has had a mild brownish discharge. On examination, she is mildly tender in the lower abdomen and bimanual examination showed cervical motion tenderness on the left. What would be the first important investigation for this patient?

A. Diagnostic laparoscopy
B. Serum β-hCG
C. Swab for both *Chlamydia trachomatis* and *Neisseria gonorrhoeae*
D. Transvaginal ultrasound scan of the pelvis
E. Urine pregnancy test

SEXUALLY TRANSMITTED INFECTIONS

60. What is the most common STI in women who are <25 years old?

A. *Chlamydia trachomatis*
B. Herpes simplex
C. Human immunodeficiency virus (HIV)
D. *Neisseria gonorrhoeae*
E. Syphilis

61. A 20-year-old student complaints of a 2-day history of painful micturition associated with lower abdominal pains and a vaginal discharge. She is examined and found to have an inflamed and swollen Bartholin's gland and a purulent urethral discharge. What is the most likely cause of her symptoms?

A. Bacterial vaginosis
B. *Chlamydia trachomatis*
C. *Neisseria gonorrhoeae*
D. *Treponema pallidum* (Syphilis)
E. *Trichomonas vaginalis*

62. A 21-year-old woman attends the emergency unit complaining of painful micturition and lower abdominal pain associated with a vaginal discharge and a mild fever. She had unprotected casual sexual intercourse a few days ago and is worried about having acquired a STI. What would be the most appropriate step to take in her management?

A. Treat with appropriate antibiotics for both *Chlamydia trachomatis* and *Neisseria gonorrhoeae* (such as ciprofloxacin) and institute contract tracing
B. Collect an midstream urine sample (MSU), urethral and high vaginal swabs for microscopy, culture and sensitivity and commence on azithromycin, and institute contract tracing
C. Collect a urethral and endocervical swab for microscopy and sensitivity and treat with a cephalosporin and institute contract tracing

D. Perform a NAAT on vulvovaginal swabs, collect swabs from the urethra and endocervix for microscopy, culture and sensitivity and commence on azithromycin, and institute contract tracing
E. Treat with azithromycin and review after 48 hours and if no response, obtain swabs from the urethra and endocervix for culture and sensitivity and institute contract tracing

63. Which STI is associated with lower genital tract cancers?
A. *Chlamydia trachomatis*
B. HPV
C. Herpes simplex
D. HIV
E. *Neisseria gonorrhoeae*

64. Which STI is most likely to cause acute urinary retention in a 20-year-old student?
A. *Chlamydia trachomatis*
B. Herpes simplex
C. HPV
D. *Neisseria gonorrhoeae*
E. *Treponema pallidum*

65. A patient has been infected with the spirochaete *Treponema pallidum*. When will this infection be labeled secondary syphilis?
A. The symptoms present for 4–6 weeks after the initial infection
B. The symptoms manifest 4–10 weeks after appearance of the chancre
C. The symptoms manifest from 6 weeks to 3 months after the initial infection
D. The symptoms manifest from 3 to 12 months after the initial infection
E. The symptoms manifest with 3 weeks of the initial infection and manifest as kissing ulcers on the vulva

66. A diagnosis of syphilis has been made on a 23-year-old who presented with kissing ulcers on her vulva. What is the treatment of choice for this patient?
A. Azithromycin
B. Benzathine penicillin
C. Cephalexin and azithromycin
D. Doxycycline
E. Erythromycin

67. What is the most common presentation of HIV infection?
A. Asymptomatic
B. Genital warts from immunodeficiency
C. Cervical and vulva pre-neoplastic lesions (high-grade squamous dysplasia)
D. Recurrent genital infections (*Candida*, HSV, and molluscum contagiosum) from immunodeficiency
E. Tuberculosis

PREMALIGNANT DISORDERS OF THE GENITAL TRACT

68. What proportion of vulva cancers are preventable?

A. 25% (1:4)
B. 33% (1:3)
C. 50% (1:2)
D. 69% (2:3)
E. 75% (3:4)

69. A woman has had cervical cancer screening and referred for colposcopy. What is the magnification of the cervix at colposcopy?

A. 2–5%
B. 5–20%
C. 10–30%
D. 20–40%
E. 30–50%

70. Which substance is applied to the cervix prior to colposcopy to help identify cells that have an increased turnover (dysplastic)?

A. 1% acetic acid
B. 5% acetic acid
C. 10% acetic acid
D. 5% Lugol's iodine
E. 10% Lugol iodine

71. In the prevention of cervical cancer, primary and secondary approaches are adopted worldwide. Which vaccination offers the most effective prevention?

A. Monovalent
B. Bivalent
C. Quadrivalent
D. Pentavalent
E. Nonvalent

BENIGN CONDITIONS OF THE VULVA

72. What is the most common symptom of benign vulva disorders?

A. Change in pigmentation
B. Discharge
C. Itching
D. Rash
E. Soreness

73. A woman presents with itching of the vulva and soreness. She is examined and a diagnosis of lichen sclerosus is made. What type of pathology is this condition?

A. A bacterial infective disorder
B. A fungal infective disorder
C. A viral infective disorder
D. An allergic dermatitis
E. An autoimmune condition

74. A 19-year-old woman attends with a painful swelling on her vulva. Following your history and examination, she is diagnosed with a right Bartholin's abscess. What is the treatment of this condition?

A. Incision and drainage and intravenous antibiotics
B. Incision and drainage and oral antibiotics

C. Intravenous antibiotics
D. Marsupialization and antibiotics
E. Oral antibiotics

75. A 30-year-old woman attends complaining of painful sexual intercourse for the past 3 years. The pain is experienced both during penetration and after—often lasting for a few hours. She says that this has been getting progressively worse. Her periods are painful especially from the 2nd to the 5th day. When examined, the lower genital tract is normal but the uterus is retroverted and of limited mobility. What is the most likely cause of her dyspareunia?

A. Adenomyosis
B. Endometriosis
C. Irritable bowel syndrome
D. PID
E. Vulvodynia

GYNECOLOGICAL ONCOLOGY

Cervical Cancer

76. Cervical cancer is one of the most common lower genital tract cancers worldwide. What is the most important risk factor for cervical cancer?

A. HPV infection
B. Immunodeficiency
C. Multiple sexual partners
D. Oral contraceptives
E. Smoking

77. Which is the most common histological type of cervical cancer?

A. Adenocarcinoma
B. Adenosquamous
C. Clear cell
D. Serous carcinoma
E. Squamous

78. A 39-year-old woman presents with a 6 weeks history of postcoital bleeding. Her last cervical cancer screening was 4 years ago and was normal. She also complaints of a brownish vaginal discharge but this is not foul smelling. When examined she is found a suspicious looking cervical lesion at 7'o clock position. What would be the most important investigation in this patient?

A. Computerized tomographic scan of the pelvis
B. Examination under anesthesia
C. Hysteroscopy and biopsy
D. MRI of the pelvis
E. Punch biopsy

79. What investigation should a patient with a diagnosis of cervical cancer have to best define spread of the disease in the pelvis?

A. Computerized tomographic scan of the pelvis
B. Examination under anesthesia

C. MRI of the pelvis
D. PET scan
E. Transabdominal ultrasound

80. What is the most common cause of death in women with cervical cancer?

A. Hemorrhage
B. Liver failure
C. Metastases to the liver
D. Renal failure
E. Sepsis

Endometrial Cancer

81. What is the most common gynecological cancer in the high-income countries?

A. Cervical
B. Endometrial
C. Ovarian
D. Vagina
E. Vulva

82. A 47-year-old obese woman whose periods have been irregular for the past 10 years had an endometrial biopsy that has been reported as atypical endometrial hyperplasia. In what proportion of patients like her will this progress to cancer if its untreated?

A. 10%
B. 15%
C. 20%
D. 25%
E. 30%

83. A 67-year-old mother of one presents with postmenopausal bleeding of 3 weeks duration. She has type II diabetes on metformin. Her BMI is 35 kg/m^2. She is not on any hormonal treatment. An ultrasound shows an endometrial thickness of 6 mm. What would be the first investigation to request for in the clinic?

A. Endometrial biopsy (with pipelle)
B. FBC
C. Hysteroscopy as an outpatient
D. MRI of the pelvic
E. CT scan of the pelvis

84. Which is the most common histological type of endometrial cancer?

A. Adenocarcinoma
B. Adenocarcinoma variant
C. Clear cell carcinoma
D. Mixed carcinoma
E. Neuroendocrine carcinoma

85. A 60-year-old has been diagnosed with well-differentiated endometrial carcinoma. What would be the recommended treatment for this patient?

A. Hysterectomy
B. Hysterectomy and bilateral salpingo-oophorectomy
C. Hysterectomy and progestogens
D. Levonorgestrel intrauterine system (Mirena)
E. Radiotherapy

Ovarian and Fallopian Tube Cancer

86. Which factor has been shown to significantly (up to 50%) reduce the risk of ovarian cancer?

A. Breastfeeding
B. Combined hormonal contraception
C. Exercises
D. NSAIDs
E. Pregnancy

87. Which is the most common symptom of ovarian cancer?

A. Abdominal pain
B. Abdominal swelling
C. Dyspepsia/mild digestive disturbances
D. Vaginal bleeding (menstrual irregularities)
E. Vague symptoms

88. Which tumor marker is raised in surface epithelial ovarian cancers?

A. Alpha-fetoprotein (AFP)
B. CA125
C. CA-19
D. hCG
E. Inhibin

89. A 43-year-old woman presented with bloatedness in her abdomen of 6 months duration. She also indicated that she was having recurrent dyspeptic symptoms. An ultrasound showed a left ovarian tumor and CA125 was raised. Her RMI (risk of malignancy index) was >300 hence she was referred to an oncologist. Following a multidisciplinary team (MDT) meeting she was offered treatment. What would be the best treatment for this patient?

A. Total abdominal hysterectomy and bilateral salpingo-oophorectomy
B. Total abdominal hysterectomy and bilateral salpingo-oophorectomy and infra-colic omentectomy
C. Total abdominal hysterectomy and bilateral salpingo-oophorectomy and infracolic omentectomy followed by chemotherapy

D. Total abdominal hysterectomy and bilateral salpingo-oophorectomy and infracolic omentectomy followed by chemoradiation
E. Total abdominal hysterectomy and bilateral salpingo-oophorectomy and infracolic omentectomy followed by radiotherapy

90. A 32-year-old teacher whose mother and sister both diagnosed with ovarian cancer had genetic screening and has been told she has the mutation *BRCA1*. What recommendation should she be given after she has completed her family?
A. Combined hormonal contraception
B. Prophylactic bilateral oophorectomy
C. Prophylactic bilateral salpingo-oophorectomy
D. Total abdominal hysterectomy and bilateral salpingo-oophorectomy
E. Regular follow-up with 6 monthly CA125

91. Which is the most common type of ovarian cancer?
A. Epithelial
B. Germ cell
C. Sex stroma
D. Sex cord
E. Metastatic

92. A 60-year-old woman presents with breathing difficulties and abdominal discomfort. CA125 is raised, an abdominal ultrasound scan shows an ovarian mass with associated ascites and a chest X-ray shows a pleural effusion. What is the most likely diagnosis?
A. Immature teratoma with chest secondaries
B. Meigs syndrome
C. Mucinous adenocarcinoma with chest secondaries
D. Non-gestational choriocarcinoma with chest secondaries
E. Serous adenocarcinoma with chest secondaries

Vulva and Vaginal Cancer

93. What histological type of vulva cancer is the most common?
A. Adenocarcinoma
B. Adenosquamous carcinoma
C. Basal cell carcinoma
D. Malignant melanoma
E. Squamous cell carcinoma

94. Which risk factor is considered the greatest with regards to vulva cancers?
A. Age
B. Autoimmune
C. Genetic predisposition
D. Immunodeficiency
E. Infection with HPV

95. What is the most common presentation of women with vulva cancer?

A. Abnormal bleeding or vaginal discharge
B. Asymptomatic
C. Pigmentated lump on the vulva
D. Ulceration of the vulva
E. Vulva itching

96. A 68-year-old woman presents with vulva itching and a small lump on the left vulva. When examined there is a lump on the left labium majorum about 3 cm from the midline. There is no lymphadenopathy. A biopsy confirms this to be squamous cell carcinoma stage 1A. What would be the treatment for this patient?

A. Chemotherapy
B. Chemoradiation
C. Radical excision and lymph node dissection
D. Radiotherapy
E. Wide excision and groin node dissection

97. What is the most common cause of death in women with vulva cancer?

A. Hemorrhage
B. Liver failure from metastasis
C. Multiple site distant metastases
D. Neurological complications including hemorrhage
E. Renal failure from metastasis

98. Which type of vagina cancer is common in young girls with a peak incidence at the age of 8 years?

A. Adenocarcinoma
B. Sarcoma botryoides
C. Secondary from nongestational choriocarcinoma
D. Secondary from ovarian cancers
E. Squamous cell carcinoma

MENOPAUSE AND HORMONE REPLACEMENT THERAPY

99. The climacteric is the period leading to cessation of menstruation. What is the average length of this period?

A. 0–1 year
B. 1–2 years
C. 2–5 years
D. 5–10 years
E. 10–15 years

100. With regard to the physiological changes that occur around menopause, which hormonal changes occur first?

A. Fall in inhibin level
B. Fall in estradiol level
C. Increase in the pulsatility of GnRH production
D. Rise in FSH level
E. Rise in LH level

101. What is the definition of premature ovarian insufficiency (POI)?

A. Onset of menopause <35 years
B. Onset of menopause <40 years
C. Onset of menopause <43 years
D. Onset of menopause <45 years
E. Onset of menopause <47 years

102. A 51-year-old woman has attended with a complaint of infrequent periods. Her last period was 4 months ago. She also complains of night sweats, being irritable, and mood swings. When will this woman be diagnosed as menopausal?

A. She has been amenorrhoeic for at least 4 months
B. She has been amenorrhoeic for at least 6 months
C. She has been amenorrhoeic for at least 12 months
D. She has a raised FSH of >30 IU/L
E. She has a raised LH of >30 IU/L

103. What would be the first treatment you will offer a 54-year-old woman who has not had a hysterectomy attends with menopausal symptoms which include night sweats, lack of energy, and irritability?

A. Combined estrogen and progestogens (continuous)
B. Complementary treatment (e.g., reflexology, hypnotism, and acupuncture)
C. Lifestyle and dietary modification
D. Estrogen tablets
E. SSRIs such a fluoxetine

104. A 53-year-old woman who suffers from severe menopausal symptoms wishes to go on hormonal therapy. What would be an absolute contraindication to this treatment?

A. Active liver disease
B. Large uterine fibroids
C. Migraine with aura
D. Past history of breast disease
E. Strong family history of venous thromboembolism (VTE)

GENITAL PROLAPSE AND UROGYNECOLOGY

105. Which is the most important ligament that supports the uterus in its normal anatomical position?

A. Pubocervical ligament
B. Puborectalis ligament
C. Round ligament
D. Transverse cervical (cardinal) ligament
E. Uterosacral ligament

106. A 65-year-old woman comes to the clinic complaining of a lump in her vagina and a dragging sensation in the lower abdomen. She has had three normal vaginal deliveries. On further questioning, she states that she has to get up at night many times to empty her bladder. When she is examined there is prolapse of the anterior vaginal wall, the posterior vaginal wall and descent of the uterus to the level of the hymenal ring. How will you classify the prolapse based on the POP-Q tool?

A. Stage I with cystocele and enterocele
B. Stage I with a cystocele and rectocele
C. Stage II with a cystocele and enterocele
D. Stage II with a cystocele and rectocele
E. Stage III with a cystocele, rectocele, and enterocele

107. A 60-year-old sexually active woman who had a hysterectomy and bilateral salpingo-oophorectomy 10 years ago attends with symptoms of genital prolapse. The notes are reviewed and it is noted that at her surgery, there were extensive adhesions that made the surgery very difficult. She is examined and found to have a vault prolapse and an anterior wall/compartment prolapse (cystocele). What would be the treatment for this patient?

A. Abdominal sacrocolpopexy
B. Anterior repair
C. Colpocleisis
D. Sacro-spinous fixation and anterior repair
E. Shelf-pessary

108. A shelf pessary has been inserted as treatment for genital prolapse in a 55-year-old postmenopausal women with stage II genital prolapse. How often should the pessary be replaced or reviewed?

A. 2 monthly
B. 2–3 monthly
C. 3–6 monthly
D. 6–9 monthly
E. 9–12 monthly

109. A 54-year-old woman has been diagnosed with vault prolapse and following counseling wishes to have surgery. What is the main advantage of the vaginal over the abdominal approach in correcting her prolapse?

A. The length of hospital stay is shorter than with the abdominal approach
B. The risk of backache is much less with an abdominal approach
C. The vaginal approach is more successful
D. The vagina maintains it anatomical position with the abdominal approach
E. Urinary incontinence is much less with the abdominal approach

110. What is the average number of times an average person empties their bladder a day?

A. 2–4
B. 4–6
C. 6–8
D. 8–10
E. 10–12

111. A 48-year-old woman complaints of urinary frequency, urgency, and urge incontinence. She is examined and there are no signs of prolapse. What would be the initial investigation to perform on this patient?

A. A 3-day bladder diary
B. Ultrasound scan of the bladder for residual urine volume after she has voided
C. Urinalysis
D. Urine culture and sensitivity
E. Urodynamics

112. A 62-year-old mother of two attends the outpatient having been referred with a 2-year history of stress urinary incontinence. She leaks when she coughs or sneezes and this is worse when she goes for her aerobic exercises. She neither has frequency nor nocturia and there is no urgency or urge incontinence. When examined her BMI is 29 kg/m^2 and there are no signs of genital prolapse. What would be the first-line management of this patient?

A. Anticholinergics such as tolterodine
B. Bladder retraining
C. Lifestyle modification consisting of fluid management and weight reduction
D. Pelvic floor exercises
E. Surgery in the form of a sling procedure

CONTRACEPTION

113. Which method of contraception prevents pregnancies mainly by interfering with implantation?

A. Combined hormonal contraception
B. Intrauterine devices
C. Lactational amenorrhea
D. Progestogen only tablets
E. Spermicides

114. What is the most effective female method of contraception?

A. Copper intrauterine device
B. Diaphragm
C. Levonorgestrel intrauterine system (Mirena)
D. Sterilization
E. Subdermal implant (Nexplanon)

115. Which WHO medical eligibility criterion (WHOMEC) is characterized by a condition for which the theoretical or proven risks of contraception outweighs the advantages of using it?

A. WHOMEC1
B. WHO MEC2
C. WHOMEC3
D. WHOMEC4
E. WHOMEC5

116. A 30-year-old woman who has never been pregnant attends for contraceptive advice. She says that her periods are regular but very heavy and she has to wear super pads. Her BM is 32 kg/m^2. There is no significant relevant medical or surgical history. Her LMP was 4 weeks ago. What would be the best method of contraception for her?

A. Combined hormonal contraception
B. Copper intrauterine device
C. Depo-Provera (depo-medroxyprogesterone acetate)
D. Levonorgestrel intrauterine system (Mirena)
E. Subdermal implant (Nexplanon)

117. Which of this is an acceptable approach to starting combined hormonal contraception?

A. Starting on days 2–3 after a normal vaginal delivery
B. Starting on days 2–4 of a regular 28–30 day menstrual cycle
C. Starting on days 3–4 after a miscarriage
D. Starting on days 5–6 after a termination of pregnancy
E. Starting on days 6–8 of an irregular 35–42 day menstrual cycle

118. Which of the following is not a noncontraceptive benefit of the combined hormonal contraception?
A. Protects against bowel cancer
B. Protects against cervical cancer
C. Protects against endometrial cancer
D. Protects against menopausal symptoms
E. Protects against ovarian cancer

119. A 20-year-old student wishes to go on an effective contraceptive. Her periods are irregular and she suffers from acne and facial hirsutism. Her BMI is 28 kg/m^2. What would be the best contraceptive for this student?
A. Combined hormonal contraception
B. Progestogen only implant (Nexplanon®)
C. Progestogen only tablets (Minipill)
D. Progesterone injection (Depo-Provera)
E. The levonorgestrel intrauterine system (Mirena®)

120. A 47-year-old woman has had the Mirena inserted for heavy menstrual bleeding and for contraception. How long will she be allowed to use the device for?
A. 3 years
B. 4 years (i.e., until the age of 50 years)
C. 5 years
D. 7 years
E. Until she has been amenorrheic for 1 year

121. A woman has just been started on the combined oral contraceptive pill. When would it be advisable for her to attend for evaluation of abnormal vaginal bleeding?
A. Any intermenstrual bleeding
B. Bleeding that is lasting more than the normal period
C. She has unscheduled vaginal bleeding after 3 months
D. Unscheduled vaginal bleeding after 6 months
E. Whenever she experiences any unscheduled vaginal bleeding

122. During counseling of a woman who has opted for an intrauterine device, what should she be told about the time when it is most likely to be expelled?
A. First 3 months
B. First 6 months
C. First 12 months
D. Last 6 months of the lifespan of the device
E. Second 12 months

123. A 36-year-old woman has been seen with a request for sterilization. She has had four normal vaginal deliveries and does not want to have more children. What failure rate should she be given for sterilization?

A. 1:100
B. 1:150
C. 1:200
D. 1:300
E. 1:500

124. What is the failure rate of vasectomy?

A. 1:200
B. 1:300
C. 1:500
D. 1:1,000
E. 1:2,000

125. A 37-year-old woman has come for emergency contraception. She had unprotected sexual intercourse 48 hours ago. Which is the best emergency contraception to give this woman?

A. Copper intrauterine device
B. Levonorgestrel (Levonelle)
C. Selective progesterone receptor modulator (Mifepristone)
D. The levonorgestrel intrauterine device (Mirena)
E. Ulipristal acetate (anti-progestogen)

PRINCIPLES OF SURGERY IN GYNECOLOGY

126. In which anatomical compartment of the abdomen should palpation for the kidneys be made?

A. Epigastric
B. Hypochondrium
C. Iliac fossae
D. Lumbar
E. Suprapubic

127. What is the main disadvantage of the Pfannenstiel incision over a midline incision in gynecological abdominal surgery?

A. Greater risk of incisional hernia
B. Increased risk of adhesions
C. Longer hospital stay with Pfannenstiel incision
D. More need for pain killers post operatively
E. Poorer/limited exposure

128. In which of these situations is the consent given for surgery not valid?

A. A 15-year-old who consents for a termination of pregnancy having declined to involve her parents
B. A 16-year-old who refuses to consult her parents consents for appendicectomy
C. A 26-year-old with learning disability who attends with her boyfriend who then gives consent for her to have a laparoscopy

D. A 29-year old who is brought into the hospital having been involved in an accident and the consultant operates on her because of severe internal bleeding
E. An 80-year-old who lives in a home attended with an abdominal mass and consents for a laparotomy

129. A 60-year-old woman had an abdominal hysterectomy and bilateral salpingo-oophorectomy 24 hours ago. During the ward round in the morning, her vital signs are reviewed and they show that her urine output over the last 24 hours was only 100 mL, her pulse is 120 pbm and her BP is 100/50 mm Hg. What is the most likely cause of her clinical picture?

A. Hemorrhage
B. Dehydration
C. Obstruction of the catheter
D. Pain requiring appropriate analgesia
E. Infection

130. A 55-year-old who had a vaginal hysterectomy 24 hours ago is reported to be tachycardic, pale, and hypotensive with no obvious vaginal bleeding. Her temperature is 37.5°C, BP 90/50 mm Hg, and pulse 110 beats per minute. She is on intravenous fluids. What would be the most appropriate step to take in the management of this patient?

A. Preform a quick general examination and send blood for a FBC and group and cross match and commence intravenous fluids
B. Arrange an urgent ultrasound scan to check if there is any intra-abdominal bleeding
C. Urgently call the senior on-call to review as she would most likely require surgery
D. Give 1 liter of intravenous fluids quickly and take blood for FBC and group and save
E. Review input-output charts urgently and correct any fluid deficit and increase fluid input
F. Commence on intravenous broad-spectrum antibiotics after taking blood for culture, FBC and group and save

131. What is the most important approach to minimizing the risk of wrong operations?

A. An operation list with patients details and procedure to be performed
B. Proper documentation in the patients notes
C. Proper labeling of the operating site
D. WHO safety check-list for surgical list on every patient
E. WHO safety check-list prior to every surgical list

WOMEN'S HEALTH

132. Human sexuality is the way people experience and express themselves sexually. Human sexuality involves:

A. Biological, phenotypical, emotional, cultural, and spiritual
B. Emotional, social, spiritual, erotic, and biological feeling
C. Erotic, biological, cultural spiritual, and emotional
D. Social, historical, spiritual, cultural, and biological feeling
E. Spiritual, social, cultural, clinical, and biological and clinical

133. Which is the most common complication of termination of pregnancy world-wide?

A. Hemorrhage
B. Incomplete removal of the products of conception
C. Perforation of the uterus
D. Sepsis
E. Trauma to the cervix

134. A 20-year-old girl has attended for a termination of pregnancy. She is counseled and this procedure will be performed medically. What should be done as part of offering this service?

A. Check her blood group and administer anti-D if she is Rh(D) negative
B. Check blood group, screen for STI, and offer appropriate contraception
C. Ensure psychological assessment and screen for STI
D. Screen for STI and treat appropriately
E. Screen for STI, treat, and discuss contraception

Part B: Answer and Explanations

1. **(B) 7 weeks.** Gonads remain undifferentiated until the seventh week when the SYR (sex-determining region) on the Y chromosome causes the gonads to develop into testes while its absence in the female and the presence of the female ovarian determining genes stimulate the development of ovaries.
2. **(C) 20 weeks.** The maximum number of primordial follicles is reached at 20 weeks (6–7 million) and thereafter start decreasing to about 1–2 million at birth and 300–400,000 at puberty.
3. **(C) Imperforate hymen.** Congenital malformations associated with obstruction to menstrual effluent will typically present with cyclical lower abdominal pain of onset at menarche. These abnormalities include an imperforate hymen, vaginal agenesis, and rudimentary horns that are not connected to the vagina. In the later cases the patients may present with normal menstruation from the other horn as well.
4. **(B) Bladder and bowel.** The uterus is anteverted in 80–85% of women and retroverted in 15–20%. Anteriorly lies the bladder and bowel, posteriorly the rectum and laterally the fallopian tubes, broad ligament and the ovaries at the top.
5. **(C) Interstitial portion.** The fallopian tube is divided into four parts—the interstitial (within the muscle), the isthmus (narrow portion next to the uterus), the ampulla (the longest part of the tube), and the fimbrial portion (surrounded by finger-like processes called fimbria)
6. **(A) The shrink in size.** The ovaries are almond shaped and in the post-menopausal period, they shrink, become smaller, contain no follicles, and the surface becomes wrinkled.
7. **(D) Dorsal position and inspection of the labia.** A gynecological examination must follow the pneumonic of IPPA (inspection, palpation, percussion, and auscultation) although percussion and auscultation are rarely required. Part of inspection involves appropriate exposure of the nine quadrants of the abdomen, inspection of the vulva with the patient in the dorsal position, a bivalve speculum to inspect the vagina and cervix with the patient in the dorsal position and inspection of the vaginal walls with a Sim's speculum with the patient in the lateral position. Exposure of the chest and inspection of the precordium is not part of a gynecological examination.
8. **(D) After inserting a speculum lubricated with gel or water.** Speculum examination is part of inspection and where samples are to be taken for microbiology, lubrication is best with water or a sterile gel that does not contain an antiseptic. The swab should be taken prior

to bimanual examination as this may contaminate the discharge and result in false positive cultures.

9. **(C) 8–9 years.** Normal puberty starts from 8 to 9 years and last for 3–4 years culminating in menstruation or menarche.
10. **(D) Ovarian estrogen producing tumor.** This girl has peripheral precocious puberty which is caused by various pathologies. As this is isolated (breast only) it is unlikely to be constitutional or central therefore the most likely cause is an estrogen producing tumor of the ovary.
11. **(E) Mullerian agenesis.** The fact that she has well-developed secondary sexual characteristics would be in keeping with an end-organ disorder. The absence of cyclical lower abdominal pain is diagnostic of either a hypoplastic or absent uterus. The cause of this is Müllerian agenesis.
12. **(C) Electrolyte and urea.** The most important investigation to perform on a newborn with ambiguous external genitalia is serum electrolytes and urea. This is because the salt-losing type of congenital adrenal hyperplasia is life-threatening if electrolyte imbalance is uncorrected. Other investigations can be instituted after this has been excluded.
13. **(A) 45XO.** These are clinical features of Turner syndrome which is 45XO. The presentation is with primary amenorrhea, short-stature, low set ears, widely spread nipples, and coarctation of the aorta.
14. **(E) Low progesterone and high estradiol leading to a preovulatory surge in LH.** Typical hormonal changes in the menstrual cycle include rising levels of estradiol in the follicular phase which in the late follicular phase have a positive feedback on the pituitary causing a surge in LH. This is enhanced by low progesterone levels.
15. **(D) 24–36 hours.** The LH surge occurs 24–36 hours prior to ovulation. LH induces luteinization of the granulosa cells in the dominant follicle resulting in progesterone production which adds to the positive feedback for LH secretion and causing a preovulatory FSH rise.
16. **(E) Low progesterone, inhibin, and estradiol levels.** Low progesterone, estradiol, and inhibin levels generate a positive feedback on the hypothalamic-pituitary axis resulting in an increase in FSH and LH production which results in the recruitment of a now cohort preantral follicles.
17. **(E) Threatened miscarriage.** The most likely diagnosis here is a threatened miscarriage. The cervical os is closed and the uterine size is in keeping with the period of amenorrhea. An ultrasound scan will confirm that the pregnancy is continuing and is viable.

18. **(D) Unexplained.** Recurrent miscarriages complicate about 1–3% of all pregnancies. The cause of recurrent miscarriages is unexplained in about 50% of cases.
19. **(D) Transvaginal ultrasound scan.** The most reliable investigation in this patient which will diagnose the type of early pregnancy complication she has is a transvaginal ultrasound scan. An abdominal ultrasound scan is not as sensitive as a transvaginal. Quantification of hCG will not help make a diagnosis. It will simply confirm that she is pregnant.
20. **(A) Expectant management.** Expectant management would be the first option in this patient. She is able to come for regular follow-up and is also clinically stable. Where the patient is unstable, then surgical evacuation would be the preferred option. Expectant management is successful in >80% of cases within 2 weeks.
21. **(B) Ectopic pregnancy.** The most likely diagnosis in this patient is an ectopic pregnancy. The lateralizing symptoms and signs, irregular periods and a dirty brown vaginal loss are all features of an ectopic pregnancy. Other findings are cervical motion tenderness.
22. **(D) She has an ectopic pregnancy that is managed surgically.** Anti-D is not indicated for spontaneous miscarriages, medically managed miscarriages, surgically managed miscarriages before 12 weeks, but should be administered to all surgically managed ectopic pregnancies and miscarriages after 12 weeks of gestation.
23. **(A) Complete molar pregnancy.** Complete molar pregnancies are diploid (46XX) and of paternal origin whereas an incomplete molar pregnancy is of paternal and maternal origin and tends to be triploid (69XXY or 69XXX). Placental site trophoblastic tumor, epithelioid trophoblastic tumor and placental site nodule are also all both of maternal and paternal origin.
24. **(C) To avoid pregnancy for 6 months from evacuation if hCG returns to normal within 56 days.** Following a complete molar pregnancy, it is recommended that pregnancy is avoided for at least 6 months from evacuation if hCG returns to normal within 56 days but if there is a delay in return to normal beyond 56 days then the delay should be timed from when the hCG levels return to normal.
25. **(A) Combined hormonal contraception.** Use of the combined hormonal contraception and the intrauterine device should be avoided following evacuation of a molar pregnancy until hCG levels have returned to normal.
26. **(B) Dietary modifications.** The management of constipation in pregnancy should be in an escalating manner starting with dietary modifications (increase fluid intake and dietary fiber) followed by

laxatives starting with bulk forming agents then osmotic laxatives if the former is not effective. The next option will be stimulant laxatives and if these fail, then suppositories and enemas can be considered.

27. **(C) She presents with vomiting that is associated with weight loss of >5%, electrolyte disturbance and dehydration.** Hyperemesis gravidarum is defined as intractable vomiting in early pregnancy (typically starting from 4 to 7 weeks) associated with weight of at least 5% of prepregnancy weight, electrolyte disturbance, and dehydration.
28. **(B) Oral cyclizine.** In the management of nausea and vomiting in pregnancy, the first option is supportive care and oral rehydration if the woman can tolerate fluids. If she cannot then antiemetics should be initiated starting with cyclizine as the first option. If this is not effective then other options can be used including prochlorperazine, promethazine, chlorpromazine, metoclopramide, ondansetron, and domperidone. Corticosteroids can be used as a last resort where all the anti-emetics have been unsuccessful.
29. **(D) Stage 4.** There are four phases of puberty—Stage 1—involving the start of breast development (thelarche), Stage 2—involving growth of the pubic and axillary hair (pubarche), Stage 3—the growth spurt, and Stage 4—onset of menstruation.
30. **(B) Constitutional.** The most common cause of precocious puberty in females is idiopathic (constitutional). This tends to be central precocity, i.e., the sequence of pubertal development is in keeping with those experiencing normal pubertal development at the right age. The cause is more likely to be pathology in males.
31. **(C) 14 years.** Delayed puberty is defined as failure to develop secondary sexual characteristics by the age of 14 years.
32. **(A) 45XO.** This girl has typical features of Turner syndrome which include short stature, webbing of the neck, wide carrying angle, and coarctation of the aorta. The gonads are streaked hence secondary sexual characteristics will not develop without exogenous estrogen.
33. **(E) Reassurance.** Precocious puberty is defined as onset before the age of 8 years in females and 9 years in males. The average age at menarche is 12.8 (8–14) years. This young girl therefore does not need any intervention other than reassurance.
34. **(E) She is aged 16 years and is yet to start menstruating.** Primary amenorrhea is defined as failure to start menstruating by the age of 16 years. However, if secondary sexual characteristics have developed, this may be considered a diagnosis at the age of 14 years.
35. **(D) Imperforate hymen with hematometra and hematocolpos.** Cyclical lower abdominal pain suggest that she is most likely menstruating but there is an obstruction to the flow of her menses.

The diagnosis is an imperforate hymen with blood in the vagina and uterus as there is a bulge (bluish-red) and a mass palpable above the pubic symphysis. If she has a vaginal agenesis or cervical stenosis, there will be no bulge on separating the labia minora.

36. **(E) Polycystic ovary syndrome (PCOS).** The clinical picture is in keeping with PCOS—hirsutism, irregular periods, and obesity. Differential diagnosis includes familiar as her mother suffers from hirsutism, adrenal and ovarian androgen-producing tumors and other medical disorders that are associated with hirsutism such as Cushing's syndrome. However, there are no features to suggest Cushing's syndrome. Although there is a family history, the presence of irregular periods and obesity support the diagnosis of PCOS which has a familiar tendency.
37. **(E) Mechanical treatment such as shaving.** Treatment of hirsutism should start with lifestyle modifications (if the patient is overweight), followed by mechanical treatment including shaving, depilation, electrolysis, and laser in an incremental approach and then medical treatment with the combined contraceptive pill such as Dianette and antiandrogens such as cyproterone acetate or eflornithine cream.
38. **(C) Clot dysmenorrhea.** Clot dysmenorrhea is the most common cause of secondary dysmenorrhea and it may be related to pathologies such as fibroids, adenomyosis, PID, or endometriosis.
39. **(C) Symptom diary for 3 months.** The diagnosis of PMS is best based on history and a symptom diary which is best kept for at least three months. Hormonal treatment may make the PMS worse.
40. **(E) Uterine fibroids.** Regular and heavy periods associated with an irregular abdominal mass arising from the pelvis and which is firm in consistency are typical of fibroids that are intramural. Where periods are irregular, the most likely type of fibroid is submucosal. In such women, other symptoms will include spasmodic pains.
41. **(A) Complete blood count (CBC).** Any patient who attends with heavy bleeding should have a FBC first. This will establish the baseline hemoglobin and help quantify the severity of the bleeding. As her mass is palpable per abdomen, she should have a transabdominal rather than a transvaginal ultrasound scan. An endometrial biopsy is indicated in those who are above the age of 40 years or have failed to respond to treatment.
42. **(A) Endometrial biopsy.** An endometrial biopsy is the most important investigation in this patient. An ultrasound scan (transvaginal) will triage her to have the biopsy or not depending on the thickness of the endometrium. A transabdominal ultrasound scan in the presence of a normal size uterus will not be very helpful.

An outpatient hysteroscopy will be the gold standard but this will have to be organized and a biopsy will be quick and provide a quicker answer.

43. **(E) 5 days.** Following ovulation, the egg survives and is fertilizable for 24 hours while the sperm survives in the genital tract for up to 5 days.
44. **(C) They have been trying for 12 months.** Primary infertility is defined as failure to conceive after 12 months of regular unprotected sexual intercourse where there has been no previous pregnancy and secondary if there has been a previous pregnancy irrespective of the outcome.
45. **(E) 30%.** 30% of infertility is caused by male factors, 30% my male facto, 20% by both male and female factors, and 10% are unexplained.
46. **(A) Advice the woman to lose weight.** The woman has clinical features of PCOS. The first approach would be for her to lose weight. It is advisable that she aims for a BMI of <30 kg/m^2. The partner should also be advised to stop smoking as this may affect the quality of the sperms.
47. **(D) Leiomyoma.** Uterine fibroids are the most common tumors of the female genital tract, affecting about 30–40% of women by the time they die.
48. **(C) Pedunculated intrauterine.** Clinical features of fibroids depend on their size and location. Most are asymptomatic. Common symptoms include those of increasing size, menstrual disorders (regular and heavy periods from submucosal and intramural), irregular vaginal bleeding and colicky lower abdominal pains (from submucosal pedunculated fibroids) and problems with pregnancy (miscarriage and infertility—mainly with large intramural and submucosal fibroids).
49. **(E) Red degeneration.** Red degeneration is the most common complication of fibroids in pregnancy and typically this presents with localized lower abdominal pain. Fibroids grow bigger and become softer in pregnancy.
50. **(B) Asymptomatic, i.e., identified incidentally.** Most fibroids are asymptomatic (40–55%) and of those that present with symptoms these vary from menstrual disorders and bulk symptoms from a growing mass and pain.
51. **(B) Hysterectomy.** Complications of myomectomy including hemorrhage, infections, injury to adjacent viscera, infertility, adhesion formation, and recurrence. Prior to signing the consent form for surgery, the patient must be counseled and accept that there is a risk of hysterectomy if the bleeding cannot be controlled.

52. **(D) Implantation theory of Sampson.** The implantation theory of Sampson was the first to be proposed to explain endometriosis and accounts for the common sites of endometriosis—the peritoneum of the pouch of Douglas and the uterosacral ligaments. The other theories explain location of endometriosis in other sites in the abdomen and also distant sites.
53. **(A) Diagnostic laparoscopy.** Although CA125 levels are raised in endometriosis, there are other pathologies that are associated with raised CA125 levels including inflammation. An MRI and ultrasound scan will easily identify endometriomas and possibly infiltrating endometriosis but is not sensitive enough for peritoneal lesions. A laparoscopy is the gold standard investigation for the diagnosis of endometriosis.
54. **(A) Combined hormonal contraception.** In young women, the treatment of choice for endometriosis is hormonal preparations. In this patient with heavy periods, the combined hormonal contraception would be the preferred option. While GnRH agonist are considered gold standard medical treatment, these are not considered first options for young patients like this one.
55. **(E) Pain that in the lower abdomen or pelvis of at least 6 months duration that is not exclusively during menstruation.** Chronic pelvic pain is defined as intermittent or constant lower abdominal or pelvic pain of at least 6 months duration not occurring exclusively with menstruation or intercourse and not associated with pregnancy.
56. **(A) Dermoid.** Germ cell tumors are the most common in the age group 5–40 years. In this category are dermoid cysts which contain tissue derived from embryonic germ layers such as skin, hair, fat, teeth, endocrine glands, and neural tissue.
57. **(D) Ovarian cyst torsion.** The history of intermittent and sudden-onset unilateral pain is suggestive of an ovarian cyst torsion. An ectopic pregnancy will not typically present with intermittent pain. Acute PID will present with lower abdominal pain which is generalized.
58. **(B) Endometrioma.** The history of CPP (characteristically lasting for a week from the start of her periods) associated with deep dyspareunia are highly suggestive of endometriosis. The appearance of the content of the cysts and its location make the diagnosis of an endometrioma most likely.
59. **(E) Urine pregnancy test.** In a young woman who is sexually active, the symptom of lower abdominal pain especially associated with irregular periods and a brownish vaginal discharge must raise the suspicion of an ectopic pregnancy. While other differentials will

include adnexal accidents such as torsion, a urine pregnancy test will ensure that further investigations of ectopic pregnancy are requested if it is positive. A transvaginal ultrasound scan would be useful once the pregnancy test has been done

60. **(A) *Chlamydia trachomatis.*** Chlamydia is the most common STI in women <25 years old. It is caused by an obligate organism known as *Chlamydia trachomatis.*
61. **(C) *Neisseria gonorrhoeae.*** A significant proportion of women with the STIs chlamydia and gonorrhea are asymptomatic. Those with symptoms present with painful micturition, bartholinitis, cervicitis and lower abdominal pain (if gonococcal) and lower abdominal and sometimes right hypochondrial pain, painful micturition, and intermenstrual or postcoital bleeding in the case of chlamydia. The clinical features of the patient above are therefore more likely secondary to *N. gonorrhoeae.*
62. **(D) Perform a NAAT on vulvovaginal swabs, collect swabs from the urethra and endocervix for microscopy, culture and sensitivity and commence on azithromycin, and institute contract tracing.** This patient has an STI and it is not uncommon for there to be a coinfection (i.e., two or more organisms involved). A quick diagnosis of these infections will be from a NAAT but culture and sensitivity is essential as it provides information on appropriateness of antibiotics. Treatment should, however, be started pending culture results. Contact tracing is critical to stop spread of the STI.
63. **(B) HPV.** Human papillomaviruses are common and although there are about 100 subtypes the most common STIs are related to subtypes 6, 11, 16, and 18. Of these, 6 and 11 and considered low-risk HPV while 16 and 18 are high risk for lower genital tract cancers especially those of the vulva, vaginal, and cervix.
64. **(B) Herpes simplex.** Herpes simplex virus when primary typically presents with painful blisters on the vulva, dysuria, fever, and rarely acute urinary retention. *Chlamydia trachomatis* very rarely may also present with urinary retention but this is much less common that from HSV.
65. **(B) The symptoms manifest 4–10 weeks after appearance of the chancre.** Syphilis is categorized into primary, secondary, and latent. Primary syphilis occurs 3 weeks after the initial infection and is cleared within 4–6 weeks; secondary syphilis manifests 4–10 weeks after initial appearance of the chancre and resolves after 1–6 months while latent syphilis manifest usually after 6 months and is further divided into early and late.

66. **(B) Benzathine penicillin.** The treatment of choice for syphilis is benzathine penicillin given as a single dose of 2.4 million units. Other options include doxycycline and ceftriaxone.
67. **(A) Asymptomatic.** Most women and men with HIV are asymptomatic with the diagnosis made from screening patients with STIs or in pregnancy as routine. Symptoms tend to be related to opportunistic organisms caused by immunodeficiency induced by the virus.
68. **(D) 69% (2:3).** Most vulva cancers are preventable and these are related to HPV infection. About 69% of vulva cancers are preventable.
69. **(B) 5–20%.** Colposcopy is examination of the cervix, vagina, and vulva under magnification. The magnification is usually 5–20 times.
70. **(B) 5% acetic acid.** 5% acetic acid is temporarily applied to the cervix prior to colposcopic examination to identify dysplastic cells (cells with increased turnover). The acetic acid coagulates the nucleoproteins within the cells with a high turnover and these appear white.
71. **(E) Nonvalent.** The nonvalent vaccine (Gardasil 9, 9vHPV) protests against 9 HPV subtypes including the low risk (6 and 11) and the high risk 16, 18, 31, 33, 45, 52, and 58.
72. **(C) Itching.** Pruritus vulvae (itching) is the most common symptom of benign vulva disorders. It is a symptom of infective, dermatological, and irritation disorders.
73. **(E) An autoimmune condition.** Lichen sclerosus affects about 1:300 women. It is an autoimmune inflammatory disorder that may present in very young as well as older women. Treatment is with topical corticosteroids such as clobetasol.
74. **(D) Marsupialization and antibiotics.** Bartholin's abscesses are typically secondary to bacterial infections—the most common of which is *Neisseria gonorrhoeae* in sexually active young patients. Incision and drainage is associated with a high recurrence, hence marsupialization and antibiotics would be the ideal treatment. A sample of the pus should be sent for culture and sensitivity as this will help identify the bacterial culprit. In most cases, oral antibiotics are adequate.
75. **(B) Endometriosis.** Painful sexual intercourse can be superficial (experienced during penetration) and deep (experienced after penetration). Superficial dyspareunia is related to factors in the vulva and vagina such as vaginismus, vulvodynia, and vaginitis, while deep dyspareunia is associated with causes such as endometriosis, adenomyosis, PID, and irritable bowel syndrome. The clinical features of the patient are in keeping with those of endometriosis.
76. **(A) HPV infection.** Over 99% of cervical cancers are preventable and these are due to infections with the high-risk HPV subtypes

(especially 16 and 18). Other risk factors include smoking, oral contraceptives, immunodeficiency, multiple sexual partners, early at age first sexual intercourse, and socioeconomic status (higher in women from the low-socioeconomic status). Most of these risk factors are associated with infections with HPV.

77. **(E) Squamous.** Squamous carcinoma of the cervix is the most common histological type—constituting about 75% of cases followed by adenocarcinoma.
78. **(E) Punch biopsy.** When a patient presents with clinical features suggestive of cervical malignancy, the most important investigation is biopsy for histological confirmation of the diagnosis. This is usually in the form of a punch. Once the diagnosis has been established other investigations like MRI to defined lateral spread and examination under anesthesia to stage and plan treatment would then be undertaken.
79. **(C) MRI of the pelvis.** Magnetic resonance imaging is the best investigation to define spread of cancer locally before treatment and after treatment the best investigation for recurrence is PET scan. Examination under anesthesia allows for clinical staging of the disease and planning treatment.
80. **(D) Renal failure.** Renal failure (typically from ureteric obstruction) is the most common cause of mortality from advanced cervical cancer. On the other hand, the most common sites of metastases are to the pelvis followed by the lungs.
81. **(B) Endometrial.** Cervical cancer is the most common gynecological cancer in low-income countries. However, in high-income countries, endometrial cancer is the most common genital tract cancer.
82. **(E) 30%.** The risk of progression of endometrial hyperplasia without atypia to cancer if untreated is <5% over 20 years while that for hyperplasia with atypia is up to 30%. Importantly, concomitant carcinoma is reported in up to 40% of cases hence the treatment of choice in the perimenopausal woman should be a hysterectomy.
83. **(A) Endometrial biopsy (with pipelle).** An endometrial biopsy is considered the gold standard for diagnosing endometrial cancer. This can either be done as an outpatient procedure with a Pipelle or at hysteroscopy. In this patient, the first step should be an endometrial biopsy with a Pipelle. If this fails then she could have a hysteroscopy. Other investigations like MRI will only help define local spread once the diagnosis has been confirmed. Although a FBC is important it is not the first important investigation in this case.
84. **(A) Adenocarcinoma.** Histologically, adenocarcinoma is the most common type of endometrial cancer. Well differentiated cancers

also have the best prognosis especially if diagnosed early with 5-year survivals of over 90% for stage 1 disease.

85. **(B) Hysterectomy and bilateral salpingo-oophorectomy.** The treatment for endometrial carcinoma is hysterectomy and bilateral salpingo-oophorectomy. Removal of the ovaries is critical as endometrial carcinoma is estrogen dependent and although the ovaries produce little estrogen after menopause, they are a source of androgens which are converted peripherally into estrogens. Additional treatment will depend on the stage of the disease. The hysterectomy can be performed laparoscopically, robotically, or via a laparotomy.
86. **(B) Combined hormonal contraception.** Of the factors that are known to reduce the risk of ovarian cancer combined hormonal contraception reduces risk by up to 50%. Other factors that reduce risk include, pregnancy, early age at first pregnancy an early menopause, breastfeeding, hysterectomy, oophorectomy, sterilization, and NSAIDs.
87. **(E) Vague symptoms.** About 66% of ovarian cancers present in the late stage (at least stage III). Most have vague and nonspecific symptoms. Symptoms include vague abdominal pains, discomfort in the abdomen, menstrual irregularities, dyspepsia/mild digestive disturbances, abdominal distension, vaginal bleeding, and respiratory symptoms.
88. **(B) CA125.** CA125 is raised in epithelial ovarian cancers (although it is also raised in noncancer pathologies such as endometriosis, PID, and alcoholic liver cirrhosis); CA19 is raised in mucinous epithelial tumors; hCG in nongestational choriocarcinoma; AFP in endodermal yolk sac tumors and inhibin in granulosa cell tumors.
89. **(C) Total abdominal hysterectomy and bilateral salpingo-oophorectomy and infracolic omentectomy followed by chemotherapy.** The treatment of choice for women with ovarian cancer is staging laparotomy, debulking (consisting of a total abdominal hysterectomy and bilateral salpingo-oophorectomy and infracolic omentectomy), and adjuvant chemotherapy for 6 months. Additional lymphadenectomy with or without bowel resection will depend on the stage of the disease.
90. **(C) Prophylactic bilateral salpingo-oophorectomy.** About 10–15% of epithelial ovarian cancers are hereditary. The mutations associated with these cancers include *BRCA1*, *BRCA2*, and hereditary nonpolyposis colorectal cancer syndrome (HNPCC). The risk of ovarian cancer is greatest with *BRCA1* (50%), 25% with *BRAC2*, and 12% with HNPCC. It is best for carriers of these mutations to have prophylactic surgery after completing their families. This should be in the form of bilateral salpingo-oophorectomy for *BRCA1* and *BRCA2* and

hysterectomy and bilateral salpingo-oophorectomy for HNPCC as this is associated with a significantly greater risk of endometrial cancer.

91. **(A) Epithelial.** Epithelial ovarian cancers make up about 80% ovarian cancers. Sex cord and stroma tumors make up 10%, germ cells make up 10% and metastatic tumors make up <1%.
92. **(B) Meigs syndrome.** The clinical features in this patient are highly suggestive of an ovarian fibroma which will cause pleural effusion and ascites. This is a benign tumor whose removal is usually followed by resolution of the pleural effusion and ascites. The raised CA125 is related to the ascites.
93. **(E) Squamous cell carcinoma.** Up to 90% of carcinomas of the vulva and squamous. Other types include malignant melanoma, basal cell carcinoma, and adenocarcinomas.
94. **(E) Infection with HPV.** About 70% of vulva cancers are preventable and these are associated with HPV infections (considered the greatest risk factor). Other risk factors include age and genetic predisposition. Like most cancers those who are immunocompromised are a slightly higher risk.
95. **(B) Asymptomatic.** Most cases of vulva cancer are asymptomatic. Symptomatic cases present with a variety of symptoms which include itching (pruritus), pain in the vulva or from metastasis, a lump or ulcer on the vulva, abnormal bleeding, or discharge and groin lumps.
96. **(E) Wide excision and groin node dissection.** The treatment for early stage vulva cancer is wide excision and groin node dissection. Adjuvant treatment will be determined by the presence of positive nodes or cancer free margins.
97. **(A) Hemorrhage.** The most common cause of mortality in cases of vulva cancer is hemorrhage secondary to erosion into the femoral artery by the tumor.
98. **(B) Sarcoma botryoides.** Vagina cancers are rare accounting for 1–2% of all gynecological cancers. About 75% of these are preventable as they are secondary to HPV infections. 90% are squamous and 8–10% are adenocarcinomas. Most vaginal cancers are secondary with only 10% being primary (i.e., arising from the vagina). The most common type of vagina cancer in young girls with a peak incidence at 8 years is sarcoma botryoides.
99. **(C) 2–5 years.** The period leading up to cessation of menstruation is known as the climacteric and it varies from 2 to 5 years.
100. **(A) Fall in inhibin level.** As menopause approaches, the number of follicles in the ovaries fall and once a critical number is reached inhibin production falls followed by a rise in the pulsatility of GnRH production. This stimulates more FSH and LH.

101. **(B) Onset of menopause <40 years.** The average age at menopause is 50–52 years. About 95% of women attain menopause between 45 and 55 years. POI (also known as premature menopause) is onset of menopause before the age of 40 years.
102. **(C) She has been amenorrhoeic for at least 12 months.** The diagnosis of menopause can be based on symptoms or biochemistry. A period of at least 12 months amenorrhea in a woman who is >50 is required to make the diagnosis and biochemically FSH level has to be >30 IU/L on two occasions at least 6 weeks apart.
103. **(C) Lifestyle and dietary modification.** In the management of menopausal symptoms, the first important step is education and counseling including support. Lifestyle and dietary modifications would be the first intervention followed by nonhormonal options and only when these have failed will hormonal options be considered.
104. **(A) Active liver disease.** Absolute contraindications to hormone replacement therapy (HRT) include suspected pregnancy, unexplained vaginal bleeding, breast or endometrial cancer, active liver disease, known current VTE or known thrombophilia, osteosclerosis, and uncontrolled hypertension. Relative contraindications include yet to be investigated AUB, past history of benign breast disease, unconfirmed personal or strong family history of VTE, chronic liver disease, migraine with aura, and large uterine fibroids.
105. **(D) Transverse cervical (cardinal) ligament.** The transverse cervical ligament is the most important ligamentous support of the normal anatomical position of the uterus. The round ligament helps maintain the uterus in its anteverted position. The other supporting structures of the pelvic organs are the muscles of the pelvic floor of which the levator ani is the most crucial.
106. **(D) Stage II with a cystocele and rectocele.** She has stage II prolapse because the descent of the uterus is to the hymenal ring but not outside but in addition, she has a descent of the anterior compartment (cystocele) and the posterior compartment (rectocele). She does not have an enterocele which is prolapse of the posterior fornix with intestines and the stage will be III if the uterus prolapses outside the hymenal ring.
107. **(D) Sacro-spinous fixation and anterior repair.** In this patient, conservative management will not be effective and neither will be ring and shelf-pessaries. The best treatment is surgery and for the vault prolapse the options are sacrospinous fixation and sacrocolpopexy. In view the difficulties with the hysterectomy, the abdominal approach (sacrocolpopexy) should be avoided. Sacrospinous fixation is therefore the surgery of choice but this will not correct the cystocele hence an

anterior repair will be required. As the woman is sexually active, a colpocleisis will be inappropriate.

108. **(C) 3–6 monthly.** Pessaries should be reviewed every 3–6 months. This is to ensure that there are no complications such as ulcerations, difficulties with sexual intercourse, stuck pessary, and vaginal discharge. At the review visits the size of the pessary should be reviewed as with time there is a need to insert smaller sizes as the supporting structures of the prolapse improve with correction.

109. **(A) The length of hospital stay is shorter than with the abdominal approach.** The two approaches to surgical treatment of vault prolapse are abdominal (sacrocolpopexy) and vaginal (sacrospinous fixation). The former is associated with prolonged hospital stay, backache, and increased risk of urinary incontinence but the vaginal length and anatomy are maintained and the success rate is higher whereas the vaginal route is associated with a shorter hospital stall, need to ness analgesia, an angled vagina making sexual intercourse uncomfortable, and a higher recurrence rate.

110. **(C) 6–8.** The average person empties their bladder six to eight times per 24 hours depending to an extent on their fluid intake.

111. **(C) Urinalysis.** For patients presenting with urinary incontinence especially those highly suggestive of detrusor overactivity, urinalysis is the first and most important investigation. Subsequent investigations will depend on whether the presence of urinary tract infections or not. If there is no infection, then a 3-day bladder diary would allow quantification and qualification of the symptoms as well as providing an insight to type and intake of fluids.

112. **(D) Pelvic floor exercises.** There are three approaches to treating women with urinary incontinence—conservative, medial, and surgery. Every woman presenting with urinary incontinence should first be offered conservative management which consists of education on fluid intake (especially for those with features of an overactive bladder), bladder training (for those with an overactive bladder), and pelvic floor exercises (for everyone). For those with stress incontinence as the only symptom, surgery in the form of cling procedures would be considered if conservative management is unsuccessful.

113. **(B) Intrauterine devices.** The mechanisms of action of contraceptives include inhibition of ovulation (combined hormonal contraception, progestogens only, and lactational amenorrhea), interruption of the journey of the gametes (sterilization), preventing implantation (intrauterine contraceptive devise), interfering with sperm viability (spermicides), and prevention of sperms being deposited in the vagina or reaching the cervical canal (condoms, diaphragms, and caps).

114. **(E) Subdermal implant (Nexplanon).** The effectiveness of contraceptives depends on how they are used. The long-acting reversible contraceptives and sterilization are the most effective because of less reliance on the user. The most effective form of female contraception is the subdermal implant (Nexplanon) (0.05%) followed by the levonorgestrel intrauterine system (0.2%). Sterilization has a failure rate of 1:200 (0.5%) compared to 0.05% for the implant, 0.2% for Mirena, and 0.8% for copper intrauterine device.
115. **(C) WHOMEC3.** There are only four eligibility criteria—WHOMEC 1 is for conditions in which there is no restriction for the use of the contraceptive method, 2 is for a condition for which the advantages of using the method generally outweigh the theoretical or proven risks, 3 is for conditions in which the theoretical or proven risks usually outweigh the advantages of using the method, and 4 are conditions for which the health risk of using the contraceptive method are unacceptable.
116. **(D) Levonorgestrel intrauterine system (Mirena).** The best contraceptive for this woman will be one which is not only effective but is able to ameliorate her heavy periods. The two options are combined hormonal contraception (which can be oral, transdermal, or vaginal) and the levonorgestrel intrauterine system (Mirena). The Mirena is a better option as it has a higher efficacy and is the treatment of choice for heavy menstrual bleeding.
117. **(B) Starting on days 2–4 of a regular 28–30 day menstrual cycle.** The best time to start combined hormonal contraception is on day 2–4 of the menstrual cycle (irrespective of whether they are regular or not), day 1–3 following a termination of pregnancy or miscarriage and 3 weeks after delivery.
118. **(B) Protects against cervical cancer.** Noncontraceptive benefits of combined hormonal contraception include protection against endometrial, bowel and ovarian cancer; however, their use increases the risk of cervical and breast cancer. The increased risk, however, falls with discontinuation.
119. **(A) Combined hormonal contraception.** This student with irregular periods, acne, and hirsutism is likely to have PCOS. The combined hormonal contraceptive would not only regularize her periods but will also help with the acne and hirsutism.
120. **(D) 7 years.** Mirena® (containing 52 mg of the progestogen levonorgestrel is licensed for use as a contraceptive for 5 years. When it is inserted in women over the age of 45 years it can be used for up to 7 years.
121. **(D) Unscheduled vaginal bleeding after 6 months.** Women who are commenced on hormonal contraception should be informed that

unscheduled bleeding is common especially in the first few months after starting the hormones. This unscheduled bleeding must be assessed and investigated if it persists after 6 months.

122. **(A) First 3 months.** Expulsion which can occur spontaneously especially in those with heavy periods occurs in about 5% of cases; the highest expulsion rate occurs in the first 3 months after insertion and thereafter falls significantly. The infection rate is also highest un the first 3 months.
123. **(C) 1:200.** The failure rate of sterilization is 1:200 (0.5%). The best time to sterilize a woman is when she is menstruating as it can be almost certain that she is not pregnant. Sterilization at other times must be done with caution and it is advisable that the woman uses an effective contraception until the next period.
124. **(E) 1:2,000.** The failure rate of vasectomy is 1:2,000, hence it is more effective than female sterilization. Furthermore, it is easy to perform and associated with fewer complications compared to female sterilization.
125. **(A) Copper intrauterine device.** The best form of emergency contraception is the copper intrauterine device. It is effective for 5 days from ovulation or 5 days after ovulation. The Mirena® and Mifepristone (RU 486) are not licensed for use as emergency contraceptives.
126. **(D) Lumbar.** The abdomen is divided into nine compartments. The kidneys are located in the lumbar regions with the right being lower than the left because of the impact of the liver on the kidney.
127. **(E) Poorer/limited exposure.** The Pfannenstiel incision is a transverse suprapubic incision used for most gynecological laparotomies. Its main advantages include, being more cosmetic, quicker recover (shorter hospital stay and less need for pain killers), lower risk of incisional hernia, and intra-abdominal adhesion formation. The mid-line incision offers better exposure, is quicker to enter the abdominal cavity, and can easily be extended but has an increased risk of incisional hernia, is less cosmetic and associated with a higher risk of adhesion formation. Hemorrhage at the time of surgery is greater with the Pfannenstiel incision.
128. **(C) A 26-year-old with learning disability who attends with her boyfriend who then gives consent for her to have a laparoscopy.** Consent if valid if it is given voluntarily by someone who has capacity or in the case of someone who does not have capacity or reached the age of maturity by someone in position of locus parentis (parent or acting in that role) or if between 14 and 16 and fulfils the Fraser criteria (understands the decision being taken and implications). A boyfriend is not a person in locus parentis and therefore cannot give valid consent for someone with learning disability.

129. **(A) Hemorrhage.** The patient's symptoms are suggestive of hypovolemia, most likely from hemorrhage. Although dehydration is a possibility a low urine output over the 24 hours is from inadequate volume replacement, this would have been addressed and furthermore fluid replacement after major surgery is usually of sufficient volume to generate more urine. An infection causing these symptoms is highly unlikely 24 hours after surgery. Pain may cause tachycardia but not oliguria.
130. **(A) Preform a quick general examination and send blood for a FBC and group and cross match and commence intravenous fluids.** The clinical picture is in keeping with hemorrhage and the most appropriate management is ensuring that an intravenous access has been secured, blood is sent for a FBC and group and cross match and a general examination to confirm that there is indeed intra-abdominal hemorrhage. Following this, the consultant or senior must be called as she is most likely to require exploratory surgery. While an ultrasound scan may help to confirm the bleeding, the diagnosis of hemorrhage in such patients should primarily be clinical.
131. **(D) WHO safety check-list for surgical list on every patient.** Wrong operations should be a "never event", i.e., should not happen. The best way to avoid this is ensuring that every member of the operating team takes responsibility for the surgery. This is done through regular MDT briefs at the beginning of the operation list, prior to operating on every patient, and after every patient's procedure has been completed.
132. **(B) Emotional, social, spiritual, erotic, and biological feeling.** Human sexuality involves biological, physical, social, spiritual, and erotic feelings. A nonjudgmental and respectful approach and attitude is considered the most basic requirement when dealing with sexual topics.
133. **(D) Sepsis.** Sepsis is the most common complication of termination of pregnancy worldwide. This is because most terminations are unsafe and sepsis is indeed the leading cause of maternal mortality worldwide.
134. **(B) Check blood group, screen for STI, and offer appropriate contraception.** Prior to termination of pregnancy, counseling, and screening for STI should be offered, contraception should be discussed and offered and the patient's blood group should be determined as if she is Rh(D) negative anti-D will have to be given.

SECTION B

OBSTETRICS

Part C: Extended Matching Questions

OBSTETRIC HISTORY AND EXAMINATION

Option list for questions 1–4

A	Bartholomew's rule	H	Perinatal mortality
B	First trimester	I	Parity
C	Gravidity	J	Naegle's rule
D	Leopold's maneuvers	K	Second trimester
E	Maternal mortality	L	Third trimester
F	Neonatal death	M	
G	Perinatal death	N	

Instructions: Match the description below with an appropriate term in the option list above. Each option may be chosen once, more than once, or not at all.

1. The period from 14 to 28 weeks of pregnancy.
2. The relationship of the size of the uterus by abdominal palpation to the gestational age of the pregnancy.
3. The steps taken in an obstetric examination that allow for the determination of size, presentation and lie.
4. The total number of pregnancies that the patient has that were at least 24 weeks irrespective of the outcome of the pregnancy.

ANTENATAL CARE

Option list for questions 5–8

A	ABO and Rh(D) status	H	Glucose tolerance test
B	Amniocentesis	I	Hemoglobin (Hb) genotype
C	Anomaly ultrasound scan	J	Quadruple test
D	Antibody check and full blood count (FBC)	K	Serology for syphilis, human immunodeficiency virus (HIV), rubella, FBC and ABO RH(D), Hb genotype and antibodies (booking bloods)
E	Biochemistry and nuchal translucency (NT) measurement	L	Ultrasound scan to measure crown-rump length (CRL)
F	Cervical length measurement	M	Urinalysis
G	Chorionic villus sampling (CVS)	N	Urine microscopy, culture, and sensitivity

Instructions: For each of these women attending the antenatal clinic, choose from the option list above the single most appropriate next investigation you will request at this time of pregnancy. Each option may be chosen once, more than once, or not at all.

5. A primigravida is now 18 weeks. Her pregnancy has been uncomplicated so far. She is yet to start feeling fetal movements. The fundal height is compatible with her gestation and the fetal heart is heard with a Sonicaid. Her BP is 130/75 mm Hg and urinalysis shows a trace of protein.
6. A multigravida obese woman whose last baby weighed 4.5 kg is now 24 weeks. She had a screening test for aneuploidy at 12 weeks and this was reported as normal. At 20 weeks she had a detailed ultrasound scan which was also reported as normal.
7. At 16 weeks, a primigravida is seen with no complaints for her routine antenatal visit. She had all the investigations when she booked for antenatal care and these were normal. Today her BP is 119/65 mm Hg and a urinalysis shows leukocytes and nitrites with a trace of protein.
8. Mrs TCA has come for her second antenatal visit at 12 weeks. Her first visit was at 9 weeks when an ultrasound scan showed a 9 week's singleton fetus. She has had no problems so far. An ultrasound today was normal.

NORMAL PHYSIOLOGY OF PREGNANCY

Option list for questions 9–11

A	Blood pressure (BP)	H	Red cell mass
B	Blood volume	I	Respiratory rate
C	Cardiac output	J	Tidal volume
D	Creatinine clearance	K	White cell count
E	Factor II	L	
F	Hear rate	M	
G	Platelet count	N	

Instructions: During pregnancy various physiological changes occur, there may be an increase, a fall, or unchanged in various variables. Changes in pregnancy are described for each of the variable described below. Choose from the option list above the best variable that follows the behavior described. Each option may be chosen once, more than once, or not at all.

9. There is a fall in the second trimester and a subsequent rise to prepregnancy levels in the third trimester.

10. Levels fall during pregnancy but reactivity increases in the second and third trimester only returning to normal by 12 weeks postdelivery.
11. It increases by 40% in nonlaboring women but further increases in labor.

FETAL GROWTH AND MONITORING

Option list for questions 12–15

A	Alcohol	**H**	High body mass index (BMI) (maternal obesity)
B	Chronic renal disease	**I**	Hypertension
C	Constitutional	**J**	Type II diabetes
D	Drugs such as cocaine	**K**	
E	Duodenal atresia	**L**	
F	Fetal infections	**M**	
G	Gestational diabetes	**N**	

Instructions: For each of these women presenting antenatally, choose from the option list above the single factor that may be responsible for the clinical presentation. Each option may be chosen once, more than once, or not at all.

12. A primigravida who whose BMI is 18 kg/m^2 is seen at 32 weeks of pregnancy for routine antenatal care. The symphysiofundal height measures 29 cm. She is sent for ultrasound scan which shows the AC and HC below the 10th centile with normal liquor volume.
13. A 32-year-old whose BMI is 40 kg/m^2 and whose pregnancy has been uncomplicated is seen in the clinic at 36 weeks of gestation. Her BP is 150/100 mm Hg and the fundal height measures 42 cm. An ultrasound scan for growth shows an abdominal circumference (AC) >95th centile, a head circumference (HC) on the 70th centile, normal liquor volume, and umbilical artery Doppler.
14. A primigravida is now 28 weeks and complaints of difficulties breathing and feeling easily tired. Her BMI at booking was 27 kg/m^2. When examined the fundal height measures 34 cm with a fluid thrill. An ultrasound scan shows a normal size male fetus with polyhydramnios.
15. The patient is known to be high risk and has been attending a joint clinic with the physician. She is now 30 weeks and the fundal height measures 27 cm. An ultrasound scan shows an AC and HC all below the 10th centile with reduced liquor volume.

Option list for questions 16–20

A	Early direct maternal mortality	H	Neonatal death rate
B	Early neonatal mortality	I	Stillbirth
C	Early indirect maternal mortality	J	Stillbirth rate
D	Late direct maternal mortality	K	
E	Late indirect maternal mortality	L	
F	Live birth	M	
G	Perinatal mortality rate	N	

Instructions: Choose from the option list a term/phrase that best fits the description given below. Each option may be chosen once, more than once or not at all.

16. The number of stillbirths per 1,000 total live and stillbirths.
17. The total number of stillbirths and early neonatal deaths per 1,000 total births (live and stillbirths)
18. The total number of deaths (in the first 28 days) per total live births.
19. Death of the mother in pregnancy or childbirth from conditions or their complications or their management that is unique to pregnancy occurring up to 42 days after delivery.
20. Death of the mother between 42 days and 1 year after birth, abortion, miscarriage, or ectopic pregnancy that results from previously existing disease or disease that developed in pregnancy not as a result of direct obstetric causes but which is aggravated by the physiological effects of pregnancy.

Option list for questions 21 and 22

A	Biophysical profile	H	Transvaginal cervical length measurement
B	Cardiotocography (CTG)	I	Ultrasound scan for fetal growth
C	Continue SFM antenatally	J	Uterine artery Doppler
D	Doppler of the ductus venosus	K	
E	Doppler of the umbilical artery	L	
F	Fetal kick chart	M	
G	Middle cerebral artery Doppler	N	

Instructions: These women present with various clinical scenarios. Choose from the option list the best test you will recommend for the woman. Each option may be chosen once, more than once, or not at all.

21. A 28-year-old primigravida is now 30 weeks pregnant. She is seen in the clinic and her BP is 130/85 mm Hg. Her urine does not show any protein and she does not have any symptoms. The fundal height measures 29 cm and the fetal heart rate is normal.

22. A G2P1, previous growth restricted baby that was delivered by cesarean section (CS) at 37 weeks is seen at 28 weeks of pregnancy for her routine antenatal care. Her BP is normal and the fundal height measures 27 cm. The fetal heart rate is normal.

PRENATAL DIAGNOSIS

Option list for questions 23–26

A	Amniocentesis	H	NT measurement
B	Anomaly ultrasound scan	I	Quadruple test
C	CVS	J	Reassurance
D	Combined NT and biochemistry	K	Refer for anomaly scan and fetal echo at 22–24 weeks
E	Cordocentesis	L	
F	Noninvasive prenatal diagnosis (NIPD)	M	
G	Noninvasive prenatal testing (NIPT)	N	

Instructions: Select from the option list above the best procedure that would be recommended for each of the women below who is attending for antenatal care. Each option may selected once more than once, or not at all.

23. A mother of two attends at 10 weeks to book for antenatal care. Her Hb genotype if HbAS and that of her husband is HbAC. Her first child has sickle cell Hb SC and she is very anxious about having another affected baby.
24. A 30-year-old has had her ultrasound scan for dating of pregnancy and the gestational age is calculated from the CRL as 12 weeks. The NT is measured at 3.5 mm (i.e., above the normal for the gestational age). The woman indicates that she would prefer not to risk losing the pregnancy but at the same time wants to know whether her baby has Down syndrome or not.
25. A 32-year-old attended for her booking ultrasound scan and was told the baby had a high NT. A blood sample was taken for the combined NT and biochemical screening for aneuploidy. The risk has been reported as 1:250.
26. A 40-year-old is now 15 weeks in her second pregnancy. Following counseling she opts for a screening test for aneuploidy understanding that because of her age, her risk of having a baby with aneuploidy is higher. She is, however, anxious about the risk of miscarriage as this pregnancy was after 3 years of trying.

Option list for questions 27–30

A	Abnormal NT	**H**	Open spina bifida
B	Anencephaly	**I**	Ventriculomegaly
C	Cystic hygroma	**J**	
D	Diaphragmatic hernia	**K**	
E	Duodenal atresia	**L**	
F	Exomphalos	**M**	
G	Gastroschisis	**N**	

Instructions: Choose from the option list above the single diagnosis for the fetal abnormality described in each of the scenarios below. Each option may be chosen once, more than once, or not at all.

27. A routine anomaly ultrasound scan is performed on a primigravida at 20 weeks' gestation. The single fetus is described to have a lemon-shaped head and a banana-shaped cerebellum with mild poly-hydramnios. There is no history of viral infection.
28. The woman who is a primigravida has attended for her routine detailed ultrasound scan at 22 weeks of gestation. The singleton fetus has a normal cranial and facial anatomy, a normal cardiac anatomy but there is an anterior abdominal wall defect covered by a membrane with the cord inserted at the apex of the sac. There are no other structural abnormalities.
29. This is a 37-year-old multiparous teacher who is now 26 weeks' gestation. An ultrasound scan was performed for reduced fetal movements and the baby was found to be appropriate for gestational age. There was a black structure (fluid-filled) in the left chest of the baby with a mediastinal shift of the heart.
30. A 27-year-old G2P1, is now 22 weeks. She is attending for a routine anomaly ultrasound scan. The scan shows a fetus with normal head measurements. The structures within the chest, abdominal, and the skeletal systems are all normal. The fetal bowel is, however, not covered and are floating freely in the amniotic cavity.

MULTIPLE PREGNANCY

Option list for questions 31–34

A	Cord entanglement	**H**	Twin-to-twin transfusion stage III
B	Normal discordant twin growth	**I**	Twin-to-twin transfusion stage IV
C	Selective fetal growth restriction	**J**	Twin-to-twin transfusion stage V
D	Twin anemia-polycythemia sequence (TAPS)	**K**	Vanishing twin
E	Twin reversal arterial perfusion sequence (TRAPS)	**L**	
F	Twin-to-twin transfusion stage I	**M**	
G	Twin-to-twin transfusion stage II	**N**	

Instructions: The following women with twin pregnancies have complications that have been identified antenatally. Choose from the option list about the best diagnosis of the complication. Each option may be chosen once, more than once, or not at all.

31. The woman is a primigravida with monochorionic/diamniotic (MC/DA) twins at 30 weeks. An ultrasound scan shows the following: Twin A—maternal left, cephalic presentation with AC and HC on the 50th centile with normal liquor volume, and umbilical and middle cerebral artery Dopplers [estimated fetal weight (EFW)—1,200 g]; twin B—maternal right, cephalic presentation with AC and HC on the 20th centile with normal liquor volume and Dopplers (EFW—1,050 g).
32. The woman aged 30 years is now 26 weeks with MC/DA twin. The fundal height is 32 cm. An ultrasound scan shows the following: Twin A—maternal left—breech presentation—AC and HC on the 60th centile, with polyhydramnios and normal Dopplers (umbilical and middle cerebral), EFW—800 g; twin B—maternal right—cephalic presentation very closed to the anterior uterine wall, AC, and HC on the 10th centile; liquor volume very minimal and bladder not seen. Umbilical artery Dopplers shows high resistance but middle cerebral artery Doppler is not abnormal.
33. The woman is a multipara at 34 weeks with MC/DA twins. An ultrasound scan shows the following: Twin A—maternal left—cephalic presentation—AC and HC on the 60th centile, EFW is 2,200 g, normal Dopplers and liquor volume; Twin B—maternal right—breech presentation, AC, and HC on the 20th centile, liquor volume is reduced but the single deepest pool is 2.5 cm EFW is 1,200 g. Umbilical artery and middle cerebral artery Dopplers—normal.

34. A 25-year-old presents at 30 weeks of gestation with reduced fetal movements. She is known to be carrying MC/MA twins. She says that the babies were very active the day before but have slowed down considerably. An ultrasound shows both babies alive but with no obvious movements.

Option list for questions 35–38

A	Allow normal vaginal delivery	J	Induction of labor at 35–37 weeks
B	Await spontaneous onset of labor	K	Induction of labor at 37–38 weeks
C	Assisted breech delivery	L	Internal cephalic version and breech extraction
D	Commence on syntocinon	M	Laser ablation of chorionic plate
E	Corticosteroids and deliver by CS	N	Middle cerebral artery Doppler
F	Elective CS at 32–34 weeks	O	Rupture membranes
G	Elective CS at 35–37 weeks	P	Serial ultrasound scan for growth
H	Elective CS at 37–38 weeks	Q	
I	External cephalic version (ECV)	R	

Instructions: In the management of the women below with twin pregnancies, choose from the list of options above the best recommendation that should be made with regards to management. Each option may be selected once, more than once, or not at all.

35. A 33-year-old attends for her routine antenatal care at 30 weeks of gestation. She is being followed up with serial growth scans as she has a MC monoamniotic twin pregnancy. The pregnancy has so far been uncomplicated.
36. A 29-year-old year with MC twin pregnancies is seen at 34 weeks of gestation with an ultrasound scan that shows that there is TTTS stage II. The first twin is presenting cephalic and the second is breech.
37. A primigravida is seen at 35 weeks of gestation with dichorionic DA twins with no complications. The first twin is cephalic and the second is breech. An ultrasound scan showed the growth velocity of both twins to be normal.
38. The woman is multiparous (two previous normal vaginal deliveries) who is now 36 weeks with dichorionic DA twins that have so far been uncomplicated. The first twin is presenting by the breech and the second if cephalic. Both are of the same size at the last ultrasound scan.

BLEEDING IN PREGNANCY—ANTEPARTUM HEMORRHAGE

Option list for questions 39–42

A	Cervical cancer	H	Placenta accreta
B	Cervical ectopy (erosion)	I	Placental previa
C	Cervicitis	J	Placenta percreta
D	Heavy show	K	Vasa previa
E	Idiopathic (unknown)	L	Varicose veins
F	Low-lying placenta	M	
G	Placental abruption	N	

Instructions: Each of the women detailed below presents with bleeding in pregnancy. Choose from the option list the most likely cause of the bleeding. Each option may be chosen once, more than once, or not at all.

39. The woman is 36-year-old in her second pregnancy. She is now 34 weeks and is on labetalol for hypertension. Her detailed ultrasound scan had been normal. She is complaining of mild abdominal pains and vaginal bleeding. The blood is dark in color. Fetal movements have slowed down. When examined, she is clinically stable but the uterus which is compatible with gestational age is slightly irritable.
40. A 30-year-old multiparous woman whose previous pregnancies were vaginal deliveries at 36 and 35 weeks of gestation comes with intermittent lower abdominal pains which radiate to her back and bleeding which is mixed with mucous at 36 weeks of gestation. Fetal movements are normal. When examined her vital signs are normal and the uterus is soft with the presenting part engaged.
41. The woman is in her second pregnancy, the first was an emergency CS at 39 weeks for breech presentation in labor. She has come with vaginal bleeding that is painless and an ultrasound shows a placenta which is about 1 cm from the internal os. The placenta appears to have penetrated into the myometrium at the level of the CS.
42. The woman is a 37-year-old multipara mother of two who comes to the emergency with vaginal bleeding at 24 weeks of gestation. The bleeding is painless and not heavy. A transabdominal ultrasound shows an anterior placenta that is 1 cm from the internal cervical os.

Option list for questions 43–45

A	Admit from 28 weeks	H	Transvaginal ultrasound scan
B	CS at 34–36 weeks	I	Ultrasound scan at 32 weeks
C	FBC	J	
D	Group and cross-match	K	
E	Group and safe	L	
F	Kleihauer test	M	
G	Speculum examination	N	

Instructions: For each of the following patients, choose from the option list above the single most important intervention/investigation you will recommend. Each option may be selected once, more than once, or not at all.

43. A primigravida had an ultrasound scan at 20 weeks and was said to have a low-lying placenta and vasa previa. She has attended at 32 weeks and these findings have been confirmed.
44. The woman has come at 36 weeks' gestation with bleeding that is painless. An ultrasound scan at 20 weeks had shown the placenta to be posterior and normally sited. She is clinically stable, with a soft uterus and cephalic presentation not engaged. A gentle speculum examination showed blood coming through a closed cervical. A FBC and group and safe have been ordered.
45. A 26-year-old G3P2 was seen at 26 weeks with spotting per vaginam. Her ultrasound scan at 20 weeks had diagnosed a placenta covering the os and being centrally located. A further scan at presentation confirms that the placenta is indeed covering the os. She has stopped bleeding and physical examination did not show anything abnormal.

HYPERTENSIVE DISORDERS OF PREGNANCY

Option list for questions 46–49

A	Acute renal failure (tubular necrosis)	H	Preeclampsia
B	Chronic renal disease	I	Pregnancy-induced (gestational) hypertension
C	Eclampsia	J	
D	Essential hypertension	K	
E	Glomeruloendotheliosis	L	
F	HELLP syndrome	M	
G	Nephrotic syndrome	N	

Instructions: For each woman described below, choose from the option list above the single most likely diagnosis. Each option may be chosen once, more than once, or not at all.

46. A 19-year-old girl presents at 36 weeks with headaches and right upper abdominal pains. Her BP on presentation is 150/110 mm Hg and urinalysis shows +++ protein. Her reflexes are brisk. Blood is collected for various investigations and plans are made to commence her on labetalol. She suddenly has a tonic-clonic seizure.
47. A 30-year-old primigravida is seen at 32 weeks of gestation for routine antenatal care. She is otherwise well. Her BP is 150/100 mm Hg and the fundal height is compatible with gestational age. Urinalysis shows nil protein, +glucose, and nil nitrites.
48. A 40-year-old who otherwise has been healthy attends to book for antenatal care at 12 weeks of gestation. She gives no relevant medical or surgical history. Her BP is 150/100 mm Hg and urinalysis was negative for protein and glucose. The BP is rechecked after 30 minutes of rest and it is still 150/100 mm Hg.
49. A 22-year-old primigravida is on admission with a high BP and protein in her urine. She was admitted 2 days ago at 32 weeks of gestation. Various investigations were ordered including a FBC, liver function test, coagulation screen and urea and electrolytes. Some of the results are back showing a platelet count of 70×10^9/L and alanine transaminase of 200 IU/L (raised).

Option list for questions 50–53

A	Elective CS at 37–38 weeks	H	Nifedipine
B	Emergency CS	I	
C	Hydralazine	J	
D	Induction of labor	K	
E	Labetalol	L	
F	Magnesium sulfate	M	
G	Methyldopa	N	

Instructions: Choose from the option list above the single best treatment/intervention you will recommend for each of these patients. Each option may be chosen once, more than once, or not at all.

50. A primigravida has been referred to the hospital by her midwife because her BP is high. It was 160/105 mm Hg in the community. The patient complaints of mild headaches on admission. Her BP is 160/110 mm Hg and her urine shows + proteinuria. Her reflexes are normal. Blood has been sent for investigations for preeclampsia.
51. A 40-year-old whose last baby was 12 years ago is admitted with high BP, headaches, and right hypochondrial and epigastric pains. She is now 34 weeks. When examined her BP is 150/100 mm Hg and her

reflexes are brisk. She is tender in the right hypochondrium. The fundal height measures 31 cm and the fetal heart rate is heard and is normal. Bloods have been sent for preeclampsia investigations and a strict input output chart commenced.

52. A primigravida who is on admission for preeclampsia on the labor ward has just had a tonic-clonic seizure. The seizure has stopped. But she is still very unstable.
53. A primigravida who is now 37 weeks is admitted with severe preeclampsia. She has been placed on magnesium sulfate as well as IV labetalol. Over the last 3 hours, she has remained stable. The cervix on vaginal examination is posterior, firm, 3 cm long and closed.

Option list for questions 54–56

A	FBC	H	Uric acid
B	Platelets	I	Urine spot protein-creatinine ratio (PCR)
C	Twenty-four hours urine collection	J	Uterine artery Doppler
D	Ultrasound scan for fetal growth and umbilical artery Doppler	K	
E	Umbilical and middle cerebral artery Doppler	L	
F	Urea and electrolytes, liver function text and coagulation screen	M	
G	Urinalysis	N	

Instructions: For each of the following patients, choose from the list of options above the single best investigation you will recommend in the first instance. Each option may be chosen once, more than once, or not all.

54. A 28-year-old primigravida was diagnosed with hypertension at 12 weeks of gestation and started on labetalol 200 mg twice a day. She then attended for her detailed ultrasound scan and the uterine artery Doppler was abnormal (positive notch and raised resistance index). She is now 28 weeks and has come for routine antenatal care. Her BP is well controlled and there is no proteinuria.
55. A primigravida is seen at 32 weeks for antenatal care and her BP is 140/95 mm Hg. Urinalysis shows ++ protein. The fetus is of appropriate size with a normal heart rate.
56. Mrs GP attends for her routine antenatal care at 28 weeks. She is 37 years old and this is her first pregnancy. Her BP is 140/90 mm Hg. The fundal height measures 29 cm and the fetal heart rate is normal. Her reflexes are normal.

DIABETES AND ENDOCRINE DISORDERS OF PREGNANCY

Option list for questions 57–60

A	Change antihypertensives and commence on folic acid	H	Renal function assessment
B	Change antihypertensive and offer contraception	I	Renal function and retinal assessment
C	Change antihypertensive and offer contraception and folic acid	J	Retinal assessment
D	Commence on folic acid 5 mg	K	Switch from metformin to insulin
E	Commence on folic acid 5 mg and aspirin	L	
F	Dietary advice for two weeks	M	
G	Measure hemoglobin A1C (HbA1C) and commence on folic acid	N	

Instructions: The following women either had diabetes or have been diagnosed with diabetes and are either wanting to become pregnant or are pregnant. For each woman, choose from the option list above the single most appropriate management recommendation to offer with regard to her medical condition. Each option may be selected once, more than once, or not at all.

57. A 29-year-old with type I diabetes on insulin comes to the prepregnancy counseling clinic for a discussion on starting to try for a baby. Her last HbA1C was 6.7% and a renal and retinal assessment done 2 months ago were normal.
58. A 30-year-old with type I diabetes on insulin comes for prepregnancy review. She had a retinal and renal assessment 10 weeks ago. She is hypertensive on labetalol.
59. A primigravida who is known to have type II diabetes and is on metformin attends to book for antenatal care at 12 weeks of gestation. She last had an assessment 6 months ago. She is well otherwise and her latest HbA1C was 7.2%.
60. A 36-year-old type I diabetic on insulin and also on the angiotensin-converting enzyme (ACE) inhibitor enalapril for her hypertension comes for prepregnancy counseling. Her BP is well controlled and her diabetes is also well controlled. The last retinal and renal assessments 2 months ago were all normal. Her latest HbA1C is 8.1%.

Option list for questions 61–65

A	Commence on half the dose of metformin and/or insulin	H	OGTT at 6–13 weeks
B	Elective CS at 37–38 weeks	I	OGTT at 24–28 weeks
C	Fasting blood glucose at 6–13 weeks	J	Revert to prepregnancy doses on metformin
D	HbA1C at 6–13 weeks	K	Start on insulin
E	Induction of labor	L	Start on metformin
F	Monitor blood glucose levels	M	Stop metformin
G	OGTT as soon as possible	N	

Instructions: For each of these women with diabetes in pregnancy, choose from the option list the single best management option. Each option may be chosen once, more than once, or not at all.

61. A primigravida is now 28 weeks. Her BMI was 37 kg/m^2 and following an OGTT she was diagnosed with gestational diabetes and referred to the dietician. Her average blood glucose values after 2 weeks are fasting 5.7 mmol/L, 2 hours postlunch 7.3 mmol/L, postlunch 7.8 mmol/L, and postdiner 8.2 mmol/L.
62. A multiparous woman was diagnosed with gestational diabetes at 24 weeks of gestation following an OGTT. Dietary advice failed to controlled her blood glucose values and she was therefore placed on metformin. She is now 32 weeks and an ultrasound scan shows a macrosomic baby and polyhydramnios. Her blood glucose levels from the last 2 days are within normal limits.
63. A primigravida who is known to have polycystic ovary syndrome (PCOS) and was diagnosed with gestational diabetes managed by diet alone had a normal vaginal delivery at 39 weeks. The baby weighed 3.6 kg.
64. A 30-year-old woman (mother of two) attends for antenatal care having been referred by the midwife because her previous babies all weighed over 4 kg. She is now 22 weeks having so far had screening for aneuploidy that was normal and a detailed ultrasound scan that was also normal.
65. A 33-year-old G2P1, who is known to have type II diabetes and was on metformin before pregnancy, had her metformin increased during pregnancy and in the last weeks had insulin added as her diabetic control was not very good. She has just had a normal vaginal delivery.

OTHER ENDOCRINE DISORDERS OF PREGNANCY

Option list for questions 66–68

A	Addison's disease	H	Pheochromocytoma and paraganglioma
B	Conn's disease	I	
C	Cushing's syndrome	J	
D	Diabetes insipidus	K	
E	Diabetes mellitus	L	
F	Hyperthyroidism	M	
G	Hypothyroidism	N	

Instructions: Choose from the option list above the most likely diagnosis for the clinical features each of these patients presents with. Each option may be selected once more than once, or not at all.

66. A 38-year-old G3P0 (three previous miscarriages) is now 14 weeks pregnant. She had been admitted and treated for excessive vomiting at 7–8 weeks. She has been suffering from palpitations, excessive sweating, and increasingly struggling to tolerate the hot weather. When examined, she is found to have a pulse of 108 bpm, and a BP of 140/60 mm Hg.
67. A 40-year-old who has been trying for a baby for the past 3 years finally got pregnant spontaneously. She attends today at 10 weeks complaining of having gained 2 kg since she became pregnant, a dry skin and constipation. When examined her BP and pulse are normal but there is a delay in her deep tendon reflexes.
68. A 38-year-old is seen at 23 weeks of gestation complaining of increasing thirst, excessive weight gain and inertia. When examined, she is found to have a moon-faced appearance, a BP of 150/100 mm Hg and multiple striae on the abdomen, the thighs and buttocks

DERMATOLOGICAL DISORDERS OF PREGNANCY

Option list for questions 69–71

A	Acne	H	Rosacea
B	Atopic eruption of pregnancy	I	Scabies
C	Ichthyosis	J	Seborrheic dermatitis
D	Intrahepatic cholestasis	K	Vitiligo
E	Pemphigoid gestationis	L	
F	Polymorphic eruption of pregnancy (PEP)	M	
G	Psoriasis	N	

Instructions: The following pregnant women present with a skin rash with or without itching. For each woman, select from the option list above the most likely diagnosis. Each option may be selected once, more than once, or not at all.

69. A mother of one comes to the emergency with a rash that has been developing over the last 1 week. She is 33 weeks of pregnant and her pregnancy has so far been uncomplicated. The rash is not itching and started around her umbilicus. It initially was red and has spread to her back and legs, hands, soles, and palms with large blisters appearing with the rash. When examined there are tense blisters over her abdomen, back, and limbs
70. A primigravida presents with itching and a rash of 1-week duration. She is now 29 weeks. The rash which started on the abdomen but strangely does not involve the area around her umbilicus has spread to her back and limbs but not the soles of her feet or her palms. She has been examined and there is an erythematous papular rash on the abdomen located within her stretch marks, her back and on her lower limbs and upper limbs.
71. A primigravida is seen at 26 weeks complaining of itching and a rash. The rash is mainly on her face, neck, trunk, and the back of her limbs. There is a strong family of similar skin symptoms in her mother and sister. When examined there are erythematous excoriated nodules and papular rashes on the skin of the face, neck, and limbs.

RESPIRATORY DISORDERS OF PREGNANCY

Option list for questions 72–74

A	Asthma	H	Pleural effusion
B	Bronchopneumonia	I	Pulmonary embolism (PE)
C	Covid-19	J	Suppurative lung disease
D	Cystic fibrosis (CF)	K	Tension pneumothorax
E	Influenza	L	
F	Lobar pneumonia	M	
G	Lung collapse	N	

Instructions: For each of these cases, choose from the option list above the most likely diagnosis. Each option may be selected once, more than once, or not at all.

72. A mother comes into the emergency at 38 weeks with chest pain, cough productive of rusty foul-smelling sputum, and a fever. When examined she is pyrexial (temperature 38.1°C), tachycardic (pulse 105 bpm), and tachypneic (respiratory rate 20 bpm). There are generalized crackles over the chest.

73. A 20-year-old delivered 3 days ago and was sent home a day after delivery. She has been referred because she is very unwell. She gives a history of nausea, vomiting fever, right-sided chest pain, and cough. Her oxygen saturation in air are 95–97%, Her temperature is 37.9°C, pulse 90 bpm and respiratory rate 19 bpm. There are localized signs in the chest—mainly in the right lower lobe where there is dullness on percussion and bronchial sounds on auscultation.
74. A woman had a normal vaginal delivery and soon after she complained of chest pain on the left side. She is apyrexial and her vital signs are normal. When examined there is tracheal deviation to the left, reduced air entry on the left but nothing else abnormal.

Option list for questions 75–77

A	Arterial blood gases	**H**	Pulse oximetry
B	Bronchial lavage for PCR	**I**	Sputum culture
C	Bronchoscopy	**J**	
D	Chest X-ray (CXR)	**K**	
E	CT scan	**L**	
F	FBC	**M**	
G	Magnetic resonance imaging (MRI)	**N**	

Instructions: Select from the list of options above the best first-line investigation you will recommend for each of these women. Each investigation may be selected one, more than once, or not at all.

75. A primigravida is seen in the emergency with symptoms of a chest infection. Following a clinical examination, there is a suspicion that she may have lobar pneumonia.
76. The multiparous woman complaints of cough, which is unproductive, chest pain, night sweats, and weight loss at 20 weeks of gestation. When examined, there are no obvious clinical signs but there is a suspicion of pulmonary tuberculosis.
77. A woman is brought to the hospital with severe breathing difficulties by her husband. She says that this was of a very sudden onset and although she has been slightly unwell (mild fever and nausea and occasional vomiting) she has only in the last hour taken a turn for the worse. When examined she is tachypneic and appears there is a suspicion of mild cyanosis.

CONNECTIVE TISSUE DISORDERS OF PREGNANCY

Option list for questions 78–81

A	Aspirin	H	Fetal echo at 20, 24, 28, and 32 weeks
B	Aspirin and low-molecular-weight heparin (LMWH) from 12 weeks until delivery	I	Induction at 37–38 weeks
C	Aspirin from 12 weeks until delivery and LMWH from now until 6 weeks postpartum	J	Induction of labor at term
D	Aspirin until delivery and LMWH until 6 weeks of postpartum	K	Manage pregnancy as normal
E	Await spontaneous onset of labor and electronic fetal monitoring in labor	L	Serial fetal growth ultrasound from 26–28 weeks
F	Check anti-Ro/La antibodies	M	
G	Elective CS at 38–39 weeks	N	

Instructions: Choose from the option list above the best advice you will give each of these women with respect to their management. Each of the options may be chosen once, more than once, or not at all.

78. A woman is seen at the booking clinic at 10 weeks and on review of her history you discover that she suffers from systemic lupus erythematosus (SLE). She is not on any medication at the moment. She stopped all her medication once she found out about the pregnancy.
79. A woman had an IUFD at 34 weeks of gestation. This is her first pregnancy. A postmortem examination of the baby showed endomyocardial elastosis.
80. A multiparous woman with rheumatoid arthritis is now 10 weeks. She was taking steroids for her rheumatic arthritis but since becoming pregnant she has stopped the treatment and her condition is much better.
81. A woman with SLE attended for an ultrasound can at 36 weeks and the baby was found to be of appropriate size but there was heart block.

CARDIAC DISORDERS IN PREGNANCY

Option list for questions 82–85

A	Aortic root dissecting aneurysm	H	Myocardial infarction
B	Aortic stenosis	I	Pulmonary hypertension
C	Cardiomyopathy	J	Pulmonary stenosis
D	Left ventricular heart failure	K	
E	Marfan syndrome	L	
F	Mitral regurgitation	M	
G	Mitral stenosis	N	

Instructions: Match the cardiac condition in each of these patients with the most appropriate option from the list above. Each option may be matched once, more than once, or not at all.

82. An autosomal dominant condition that involves connective tissues abnormality that leads to valvular disorders especially mitral valve prolapse and aortic regurgitation or dissection.
83. A 40-year-old primigravida presents with breathlessness, at rest and when exercising, chest pressure and pain and swollen legs. Physical examination shows pulmonary congestion, cardiomegaly, hepatomegaly, edema, and ascites.
84. A 23-year-old primigravida is seen at 10 weeks complaining of chest pain and left arm discomfort. She is tachycardic and the ECG shows a prolonged ST-segment. Serum troponin levels are elevated.
85. A 40-year-old complaints of a sudden-onset epigastric pain radiating to the back and in between the shoulder blades at 10 weeks of gestation. She is sweating and tachycardic on examination and there is a pulsating mass in the epigastrium.

RENAL DISORDERS OF PREGNANCY

Option list for questions 86–89

A	Change antihypertensive treatment	H	Serial growth scan
B	Commence on antibiotics	I	Switch ACE inhibitor, commence on 5 mg folic acid, and contraception
C	Commence on aspirin from 12 weeks	J	Urine culture and start antibiotics
D	Delay pregnancy for 6–12 months	K	
E	Monitor renal function monthly	L	
F	Renal ultrasound scan	M	
G	Screen for GDM by OGTT at 24–28 weeks	N	

Instructions: The following women are either attending the prepregnancy clinic for counseling on the basis of renal disorders or are pregnant with various complications of the renal system. For each woman, choose from the option list above the single best step you will take with respect to the management of the patient. Each option may be chosen once, more than once, or not at all.

86. A 38-year-old who had renal transplant 6 months age attends for prepregnancy counseling. She is on 20 mg of prednisolone per day. Her BP is 150/100 mm Hg and she has +++ proteinuria.
87. The woman is now 30 weeks of pregnant and is attending with the third episode of pyelonephritis. On the previous two occasions, *Pseudomonas* was isolated and treated. A urine sample has been sent for culture and antibiotics commenced.

88. A woman who had renal transplant 18 months ago attends for antenatal care at 20 weeks. Her renal function is normal as well as her BP. She is on labetalol 200 mg BD and aspirin which she started at 12 weeks. A fetal anomaly ultrasound scan is reported as normal and a follow-up growth scan has been arranged for 24 weeks.
89. A 38-year-old attends for counseling as she wishes to start a family. She had a kidney transplant 12 months ago. Her medications include ramipril (an ACE inhibitor) and azathioprine. Her BP today is 135/80 mm Hg, proteinuria is trace and her serum creatinine is normal.

INFECTIONS IN PREGNANCY

Option list for questions 90–101

A	Chickenpox (varicella zoster)	K	Malaria
B	*Chlamydia trachomatis*	L	*Neisseria gonorrhoeae*
C	Coronavirus	M	Parvovirus B-19
D	Cytomegalovirus (CMV)	N	Rubella
E	*Group B haemolytic streptococcus*	O	Syphilis
F	Hepatitis	P	*Toxoplasma gondii*
G	Herpes simplex	Q	Tuberculosis
H	HIV	R	Zika virus
I	Influenza	S	
J	*Listeria monocytogenes*	T	

Instructions: For each of these women presenting with features of infections in pregnancy, choose from the option list above the most likely infection. Each option may be chosen once, more than once, or not at all.

90. A mother comes to the clinic saying that she had experienced mild fever, malaise, and flu-like symptoms about 8 weeks ago. She was then 10 weeks. She took paracetamol and got better. She has cats at home and manages the litter. She is sent for an ultrasound scan which shows ventriculomegaly and calcifications in the liver and the brain. Fetal growth is normal as well as the rest of its anatomy.
91. An ultrasound is performed at 26 weeks on a G2P1, woman and the baby is found to have microcephaly, intracranial calcifications, and hepatomegaly. Fetal measurements are consistent with 23 weeks (i.e., there is fetal growth restriction). She gives a history of flu-like symptoms when she was about 8 weeks.
92. A 30-year-old comes to the emergency complaining of a painless ulcer on the vulva of 2 weeks. These ulcers are symmetrical on both labia majora are associated with mild inguinal lymphadenopathy.
93. A multiparous woman from the inner city presents with unproductive cough of 3 weeks duration at 28 weeks of gestation. The cough is

associated with night sweats and generalized weakness. She confirms that there are many of them in the household and her parents who have been coughing recently came from India.

94. The woman is a primary school teacher who complaints of feeling unwell for the past week. Her symptoms included mild fever, body aches, headaches, and muscle pains. Two children in her class had fever which was accompanied by red cheeks.
95. A 23-year-old primigravida attends with a generalized maculopapular rash on the trunk. She had been feeling unwell with generalized body aches, malaise, and headaches. She is a nursery assistant and says that her mother cannot recall her having any rash illness as a child.
96. The baby was born by ventouse a week ago and now presents with a purulent discharge in its eyes which are red and sticky
97. A neonate is seen with sticky eyes at 2 days of life. The mother does not recall having any obvious infection in her genital tract although she had experienced a burning sensation during micturition 2 weeks before she delivered but as this cleared on its own she never bothered.
98. A 21-year-old who is 30 weeks pregnant and recently returned from West Africa has come into the emergency with fever which is worse in the evening, body aches, and headaches. When she has the fever she shivers and sweats.
99. Mrs DMS is now 14 weeks. She confirms using drugs (recreational including injections). Her partner an IV drug user is from South Africa. A blood test shows a low CD4+ count.
100. A woman who is 36 weeks pregnant attends with an unproductive cough, fever, muscle aches, and joint pains. She has lost her taste and smell in the last few days. A CT of the chest shows a ground-glass pneumonia.
101. A 19-year-old primigravida attends at 16 weeks of gestation in acute urinary retention. She says that she has had very painful blisters on her vulva for the past 24 hours associated with pain passing urine. She has a low-grade fever and slightly enlarged inguinofemoral lymph nodes.

Option list for questions 102–105

A	Aciclovir 400 mg tds	**H**	Rifampicin and isoniazid
B	Allow normal vaginal delivery	**I**	Rifampicin, streptomycin, and isoniazid
C	Ampicillin	**J**	Streptomycin
D	Crystalline penicillin	**K**	Varicella zoster IgG to the baby
E	Elective CS	**L**	
F	Growth scan	**M**	
G	Induction of labor	**N**	

Instructions: These women have been diagnosed with infections in pregnancy. For each woman, select from the list of options above the most appropriate treatment you will recommend. Each option may be chosen once, more than once, or not at all.

102. A G2P1, previous preterm labor has been screened at 27 weeks and found to have group B Streptococcus (GBS). Pregnancy has been uncomplicated so far.
103. A mother of three who had been seen with a history of chronic cough was investigated by bronchial lavage for PCR and this has confirmed that she has pulmonary tuberculosis.
104. A woman who developed a rash 3 days ago and was informed yesterday that this was chickenpox has just had a normal vaginal delivery. As she presented >48 hours after the rash had appeared, she was not given aciclovir.
105. A diagnosis of nonprimary first episode HSV type 2 infection has been diagnosed in a primigravida at 30 weeks of gestation.

PSYCHIATRIC DISORDERS IN PREGNANCY

Option list for questions 106–108

A	Admit into mother and baby unit for therapy	**H**	Supportive therapy
B	Anxiolytics and supportive therapy	**I**	Tricyclic antidepressants (e.g., imipramine)
C	Electroconvulsive therapy	**J**	
D	Lithium carbonate	**K**	
E	Progestogens (oral)	**L**	
F	Psychotherapy and antidepressants	**M**	
G	Reassurance	**N**	

Instructions: Choose from the option list above the single most appropriate treatment for each of these women presenting with postpartum psychiatric disorders. Each option may be chosen once, more than once, or not at all.

106. The woman is 20 years old and is 3 days postpartum. She complaints of being tired, irritable, and struggling to concentrate. She is breastfeeding and the baby feeds every 3–4 hours. She does not have any negative feelings toward the baby.
107. The woman is 30 years old and is now 4 weeks post a forceps delivery. She had labored for 16 hours and developed an infection of her perineum which required antibiotics for 7 days. She now presents with a lack of interest in the baby (blaming the baby for her sore perineum),

lack of energy, loss of enjoyment of being a mother, and very little interest in the baby. She feels hopeless and fears being a very bad mother and this causes restlessness and panic attacks.

108. A 28-year-old woman who had her second baby 3 weeks has been brought in by her husband very concerned about her mental state. He says that she is restless, agitated, and exhibit confusion and disorientation. She hallucinates and sometimes talks about protecting the baby from people wanting to harm him. Sometimes she becomes so active it is difficult to slow her down. Of note is a history of postpartum psychosis after her first pregnancy. She was admitted into hospital and treated for 1 week.

MATERNAL COLLAPSE IN PREGNANCY

Option list for questions 109–113

A	Amniotic fluid embolism	**H**	Myocardial infarction
B	Anaphylaxis	**I**	PE
C	Aortic dissection	**J**	Sepsis
D	Cardiomyopathy	**K**	Tension pneumothorax
E	Drugs (magnesium sulfate)	**L**	Toxicity (drug)
F	Hemorrhage	**M**	
G	Hypoglycemia	**N**	

Instructions: The following women have collapsed either during pregnancy, intrapartum, or postpartum. Choose from the option list above the single most likely cause of the collapse. Each option may be chosen once more than once, or not at all.

109. The woman is 23 years old and had a normal delivery. Her episiotomy was being repaired when she started twitching and collapsed. She had been given a local anesthetic for the repair.

110. A primigravida is seen at 37 weeks of gestation with chest pain and left shoulder aches. She was being assessed when she collapsed and a blood test showed raised troponin levels. An ECG showed and inverted ST segment.

111. The woman is brought to the emergency by ambulance having collapsed in the shopping mall. She is 27 weeks and complaints of headaches, feeling flushed, and nauseous. She gives a history of draining water from the vagina about 3 days previously. Her temperature is 38.5°C, BP 100/50 mm Hg, and pulse is 110 bpm. She is warm peripherally.

112. A primigravida is undergoing an elective CS at 39 weeks for breech presentation. The baby has been delivered and the surgeon notes

that the blood is not clotting easily. The anesthetist also complaints that the patient has been complaining of sudden chest pain and is desaturating.

113. A 36-year-old who had been complaining of swollen legs in the last weeks of her pregnancy collapses suddenly after a normal vaginal delivery. She had complaint of chest pain and difficulties breathing before collapsing. Her oxygen saturations have fallen to 90%.

INTRAUTERINE FETAL DEATH

Option list for questions 114–116

A	Antiphospholipid syndrome (APS)	H	Syphilis
B	Chorioamnionitis	I	SLE
C	Gestational diabetes	J	
D	Hypothyroidism	K	
E	Lethal fetomaternal hemorrhage	L	
F	Obstetric cholestasis	M	
G	Rhesus isoimmunization	N	

Instructions: The following women present with IUFD at various gestational ages. Various investigations have been requested for each woman. Choose from the option list above the single most likely cause of the IUFD based the investigations performed on their results. Each option may be chosen once, more than once, or not at all.

114. The patient is a primigravida presents at 34 weeks with abdominal pain and absent fetal movements for 12 hours. When examined the uterus is compatible with gestational age and is neither tender nor irritable. She is Rhesus (D) negative and during pregnancy no antibodies were present in her blood. A Kleihauer test was positive.

115. A 32-year-old had an IUFD at 32 weeks of gestation. She had come to the clinic for routine antenatal care and the fetal heart could not be heard in the clinic. An IUFD was confirmed on ultrasound scan and following delivery a postmortem examination of the fetus showed endomyocardial elastosis.

116. The woman is 28-year-old and had seen her midwife at 36 weeks when she was told the baby was large and the water around it was excessive. She came in 2 days ago with absent fetal movements and an intrauterine device (IUD) was confirmed on ultrasound scan. Labor was induced and at delivery there was severe shoulder dystocia. The baby who is macerated weighs 4.8 kg.

PRETERM LABOR AND PREMATURE RUPTURE OF FETAL MEMBRANES

Option list for questions 117–123

A	CS (emergency CS)	**J**	Partus™ test (actim partus test)
B	Cervical cerclage and 14–16 weeks	**K**	Remove cerclage at 37–38 weeks
C	Corticosteroids and erythromycin	**L**	Rescue cerclage
D	Corticosteroids, erythromycin, and tocolysis	**M**	Speculum examination
E	Corticosteroids, tocolysis, and magnesium sulfate	**N**	Transvaginal cervical assessment
F	Expectant management and induce labor after 24–48 hours	**O**	Vital signs and complete blood count (CBC) twice weekly
G	Induction of labor	**P**	
H	Monitor vital signs 4 hours		
I	Oncofetal fibronectin		

Instructions: The following women present either to the clinic or to the emergency with various complications of pregnancy that are related to preterm birth. For each woman choose the single best treatment/next investigation you will recommend. Each option may be selected once, more than once, or not at all.

117. A 32-year-old primigravida attends at 28 weeks contracting 2–3 in 10 minutes for the past 3 hours. Her pregnancy had been uncomplicated up to now. Her vital signs are stable and speculum examination shows a short cervix (70% effaced) with a closed os. Urinalysis is negative and a CBC is sent to the lab.
118. A 22-year-old G2P0 previous termination of pregnancy at 26 weeks attends with a history of sudden gush of water from the vagina. She is apyrexial and vital signs are stable. The fetus is breech and the heart rate is normal.
119. A 40-year-old primigravida who had a cone biopsy for CINIII attends to book for antenatal care at 10 weeks. She is well and vital signs are normal. A dating ultrasound confirms the gestational age. She has been counseled and opts for a combined NT and biochemical screening at 12–13 weeks.
120. A 31-year-old presents at 36 weeks of gestation with rupture of membranes but no contractions. The fetus is cephalic with a normal heart rate. A speculum examination confirms leakage of liquor. A CBC is performed and this is normal.
121. A 30-year-old had an interval cervical cerclage inserted abdominally 3 years ago. She is now 34 weeks and presents with abdominal pains and vaginal bleeding.

122. A woman in her third pregnancy presents at 20 weeks complaining that she has been feeling heavy in her lower abdomen. Her previous two pregnancies were normal vaginal deliveries at 35 and 36 weeks. A CTG shows minimal uterine activities. On speculum examination, the membranes are bulging through a cervix that is 2 cm dilated.
123. You see a 29-year-old G2P1 who had a cervical cerclage at 22 weeks because of a short cervix at 36 weeks of gestation for routine antenatal care. She is well and the fetus which is cephalic is of normal size. Her BP is normal and urinalysis is negative for protein and leukocytes.

HEMATOLOGICAL DISORDERS OF PREGNANCY

Option list for questions 124–126

A	CXR	H	Echocardiography
B	Pulse oximetry	I	ECG
C	Compression duplex Doppler of the leg	J	Arterial blood gases
D	Ventilation perfusion (V/Q) scan	K	
E	Computerized tomographic pulmonary angiography (CTPA)	L	
F	D-dimers	M	
G	Magnetic resonance venography	N	

Instructions: For each of these women with suspected VTE in pregnancy, choose from the list of options above the single next important investigation you will recommend to help confirm the diagnosis. Each option may be chosen once, more than once, or not at all.

124. A 40-year-old obese primigravida attends with a complaint of pain and swelling in her left leg. She noticed the swelling yesterday. The foot and leg are swollen and tender on examination. She is mildly pyrexial (temperature 37.8°C). You suspect that she may have a deep vein thrombosis (DVT).
125. You see a 38-year-old grand multipara in the Obstetric Triage with sudden-onset chest pain and difficulties breathing. She gives a history of pain in her pelvis and her buttocks for the past 1 week. From physical examination and oxygen saturations, it is suspected that she may have PE but this requires confirmation.
126. A 29-year-old is admitted with cough chest pain and difficulties breathing. Her oxygen saturations in air vary between 90 and 93%. She says that a week ago she developed a swollen and mildly painful left leg. She is found on examination to be pyrexial (temperature 37.7°C), tachycardic (pulse 108 bpm), and her BP is 150/65 mm Hg. The left leg is swollen, warm, and red. She is thought to have a PE.

Option list for questions 127–133

A	Aspirin	H	Prophylactic LMWH antenatally until 6 weeks after delivery
B	Avoid combined hormonal contraception	I	Prophylactic LMWH for 10 days
C	Avoid (omit) heparin for 12 hours	J	Prophylactic LMWH from 6 weeks
D	Avoid (omit) heparin for 24 hours	K	Prophylactic LMWH from 28 weeks until 6 weeks after delivery
E	Full anticoagulation with LMWH	L	Recommence LMWH 4 hours after removing the catheter
F	Full anticoagulation with unfractionated heparin	M	Warfarin sodium
G	Omit the next does of LMWH	N	

Instructions: Each of these women requires management of either their risk of VTE in pregnancy or of a suspicion or confirmed VTE. Choose from the option list above the single most appropriate management option with regard to therapy/thromboprophylaxis for the patient. Each option may be selected once, more than once, or not at all.

127. The woman is a multipara at 40 weeks of gestation presenting with a swollen right calf. Physical examination and investigations confirm this to be a deep venous thrombosis.
128. A 25-year-old is admitted with clinical features of PE at 30 weeks of gestation. A CXR was normal and a V/Q scan confirmed the diagnosis.
129. A primigravida who was diagnosed with a left DVT and is fully anticoagulated is now 38 weeks of gestation. Her fetus is presenting by the breech and following counseling she has opted for an elective CS which is scheduled for 39 weeks.
130. The woman is a primigravida on LMWH as thromboprophylaxis on the basis of several risk factors which include her age, high BMI, an in vitro fertilization (IVF) pregnancy and a family history of VTE. She is now 41 weeks and is being booked for induction of labor in 6 days.
131. A 36-year-old presents to book for antenatal care and gives a history of two DVTs in the past. The first was when she went on the combined contraceptive pill and the second was in at the tail end of her last pregnancy which was 8 years ago. Her BMI is 28 kg/m^2 and she does not smoke. She is fit and active.
132. A 36-year-old G4P3 books for antenatal care at 10 weeks of gestation. She smokes 10 cigarettes per day and her BMI is 35 kg/m^2. She is otherwise healthy.

133. A patient who was placed on LMWH antenatally as thromboprophylaxis has just had an elective CS under an epidural. The procedure was uncomplicated and the estimated blood loss was 800 mL.

ABDOMINAL PAIN IN PREGNANCY

Option list for questions 134–140

A	Acute appendicitis	I	Labor
B	Acute cholecystitis	J	Ovarian torsion
C	Acute pancreatitis	K	Peptic ulcer disease
D	Bowel obstruction	L	Placental abruption
E	Chorioamnionitis	M	Pyelonephritis
F	Degenerating fibroid	N	Reflux esophagitis
G	Dissecting aneurysm of the aorta	O	Symphysis pubic dysfunction
H	Hiatus hernia	P	Ureteric colic

Instructions: The following patients present with the symptoms of abdominal pain in pregnancy. For each woman choose from the option list above the most likely cause of the pain. Each option may be selected once, more than once, or not at all.

134. A 24-year-old has come to the emergency at 14 weeks of gestation with lower abdominal pain of 2 days duration. The pain which started in the suprapubic region is now mainly in the right lumbar region. She has nausea and vomited once. Her temperature is 38°C, the uterus is 14 weeks size, and there is tenderness in the right iliac fossa.

135. A 20-year-old primigravida presents at 34 weeks of gestation with intermittent pain of 3 hours duration. The pain is so severe that she has had to take paracetamol. The pains are in her lower abdomen and radiate to the back. She has been passing urine more frequently but there is no burning sensation with voiding. She vomited once today when the pain was severe. Fetal movements are normal. On examination, she is afebrile and vital signs and normal. The uterus is 36 weeks in size and the fetus is longitudinal and cephalic with the head engaged.

136. A 32-year-old Nigeria in her first pregnancy has been suffering from recurrent abdominal pain since she was 10 weeks. On every occasion, the pain has been constant, and localized in the center of the abdomen. There has never been any associated nausea, vomiting, or fever. She is examined and found to be afebrile, clinically stable with normal vital signs and a gravid uterus of 14 weeks size. There is tenderness to the right of the uterus over a soft mass that appears to be contiguous with the uterus.

137. A 40-year-old multiparous woman comes to the emergency unit complaining of severe right upper abdominal pain, nausea, and vomiting of 3 days duration. The pain which is colicky is worse after meals. There is associated nausea but no vomiting. She is afebrile on clinical examination with tenderness in the right hypogastrium and positive Murphy's sign.
138. A 21-year-old presents with abdominal pain, fever, and rigors pain started 2 days ago but has got worse over the last 24 h... She has vomited twice. Her urine is dark in color. On examination, she has a temperature of 38.5°C, a gravid uterus of 28 weeks (compatible with gestation) and tenderness over the lumbar region. Her urine is dark red and there are leukocytes, nitrites, and red cells on urinalysis.
139. A 30-year-old presents with acute upper abdominal pain radiating to the back of 2 days duration. The pain is worse after eating. There is associated nausea, vomiting, and a fever. On examination, she is febrile (temperature 38.0°C), tachycardic (pulse 104 bpm), and mildly jaundiced. The uterus is 20 weeks size and there is tenderness on deep palpation just above the umbilicus.
140. A 27-year-old G3P2 has been referred to the Obstetrics Triage of the unit with a complaint of generalized abdominal pains and reduced fetal movements. She also complaints of feeling hot and sweaty more than usual. There is no history of leakage of water from the vagina. When examined she is mildly febrile (temperature 37.6°C), pulse 96 bpm and respiratory rate 24 bpm. The uterus is 32 weeks in size but is irritable on palpation and there is tenderness. A CTG shows a baseline heart rate of 170 bpm with a poor baseline variability and occasional decelerations but no accelerations.

INDUCTION OF LABOR

Option list for questions 141–145

A	Artificial rupture of membranes (ARM)	H	Subcutaneous (SC) terbutaline
B	Commence on syntocinon	I	Uterine hyperstimulation (tachysystole)
C	Emergency CS	J	Uterine rupture
D	Fill the bladder with saline	K	
E	Laparotomy	L	
F	Stop syntocinon and administer SC terbutaline	M	
G	Stop syntocinon and proceed to emergency CS	N	

Instructions: These women are being induced and have developed a complication of the induction. For each woman choose the correct action to take to manage the patient. Each option may be chosen once, more than once, or not at all.

141. Prostaglandin pessaries were inserted into the vaginal of a primigravida at 42 weeks for induction of labor. About 10 hours after, she is assessed and the Bishop score is 8 but she is not contracting regularly.
142. The woman is G2P0, undergoing induction at 38 weeks for small for gestational age. She had a second prostaglandin gel inserted 2 hours ago. She is now contracting at a rate of 6–7 contractions every 10 minutes, each lasting for 30–45 seconds. Each of the contractions is associated with early decelerations.
143. A primigravida is being induced for postdates at 42 weeks. She had prostaglandin gel followed by artificial rupture of fetal membranes and now is on syntocinon. The fetal heart rate baseline has risen from 140 bpm to 160 bpm and there are now late decelerations with reduced baseline variability for the last 30 minutes. The cervix was 2 cm at vaginal examination.
144. A multiparous woman who is being induced had prostaglandin gel 4 hours ago. She has been contracting for the past 2 hours and the contractions have been increasing in frequency. She has just ruptured membranes and the fetal heart rate is now showing a persistent bradycardia.
145. A primigravida aged 26 years is being induced for gestational diabetes that is well controlled at 39 weeks of gestation. She has had two prostaglandin pessaries followed by artificial rupture of fetal membranes. The membranes were ruptured 4 hours ago (at a time when she was contracting 3–4/10 minutes) when she was 4 cm dilated. She has just been examined and the cervix is now 5 cm dilated. She is contracting at the rate of 3–4/10 minutes.

NORMAL LABOR

Option list for questions 146–148

A	Left occipitoanterior (LOA)	**I**	Right occipitoposterior (ROP)
B	Left occipitoposterior (LOP)	**J**	Right occipitotransverse (ROT)
C	Left occipitotransverse (LOT)	**K**	Sacroanterior
D	Mentoanterior (MA)	**L**	Sacrolateral
E	Mentoposterior (MP)	**M**	Sacroposterior
F	Occipitoanterior (OA)	**N**	
G	Occipitoposterior (OP)	**O**	
H	Right occipitoanterior (ROA)	**P**	

Instructions: Identify using the list of options above the single best term/phrase that defines the position of the presenting part of the fetus. Each option may be selected once, more than once, or not at all.

146. A vaginal examination is performed on a primigravida who is in labor at 39 weeks of gestation. The cervix is 7 cm dilated and the vertex is at the level of the spines. The anterior fontanel is felt just posterior to the pubis and the sagittal suture is in the midline with the posterior fontanel around 6 o'clock.
147. The multigravida is now fully dilated with the head at the spines. The sagittal suture is across with the anterior fontanels at 3 o'clock and the posterior fontanels at 9 o'clock position. There are 2+ of molding and ++ caput.
148. A primigravida is being induced for gestational diabetes. She is having syntocinon and contracting well. She is examined and is 8 cm dilated. The vertex is at 0+1 with the sagittal suture in an oblique direction and the posterior fontanelle at 11 o'clock with +caput and + molding.

Option list for questions 149–153

A	Active second stage	H	Latent phase
B	Caput formation	I	Molding
C	Descent	J	Restitution
D	Effacement	K	Station
E	Engagement	L	Third stage
F	Extension	M	
G	External rotation	N	
H	Flexion		

Instructions: These patients are at various stages of normal labor. For each patient choose from the option list above the single best description of the phase of labor the patient is going through. Each option may be chosen once, more than once, or not at all.

149. The process in which the head of a well-flexed fetus in labor escapes underneath the pubic symphysis.
150. The process in which there is a slight rotation of the head soon after delivery to become aligned with the shoulders which have by now entered to pelvis in an oblique position.
151. The process in which the bones of the fetal head overlap each other as it navigates through the pelvis. The degree varies from the bones touching, overlapping but separable and overlapping but not separable.

152. The period from onset of uterine contractions to cervical dilatation of 4 cm. During this time, the cervix becomes effaced and there may be a show.
153. A primigravida who is in labor has been fully dilated for 2 hours and now has the urge to push and is being encouraged to bear down.

Option list for questions 154–160

A	ARM	**H**	IV syntocinon
B	ARM and IV syntocinon	**I**	Mathew Duncan's technique
C	Commence pushing	**J**	Massage uterine contractions
D	Empty the bladder	**K**	Operative vaginal delivery
E	Emergency CS	**L**	Reassess in 4 hours
F	Examination under anesthesia	**M**	
G	Fetal blood sample	**N**	

Instructions: These women are in labor. For each woman, choose from the option list above the next action to take in their management. Each option may be selected once, more than once, or not at all.

154. A multiparous woman was admitted in spontaneous labor at 39 weeks of gestation. The cervix was 5 cm dilated and the fetal heart rate was normal. 4 hours later the cervix is 5 cm and fully effaced with intact fetal membranes.
155. A primigravida is being induced at 41 weeks for postdates. She was given prostaglandin E2 gel and 12 hours later started contacting. The cervix was examined and was 3 cm dilated. 4 hours later it had dilated to 4 cm. An artificial rupture of fetal membranes was therefore performed. It has been 2 hours since the ARM and she is contracting at a rate of 2–3 contractions in 20 minutes, each lasting 15–30 minutes.
156. A multiparous woman is in the late first stage of labor and the fetal heart rate has been abnormal for the last 15 minutes as evidence by reduced baseline variability (<5 bpm), late decelerations and an increase in baseline from 146 to 160 bpm. She ruptured membranes spontaneously 3 hours before contractions started.
157. A primigravida in labor has been reported to be having persistent late decelerations at 5 cm. The vertex is 1 cm above the ischial spines in the occipitotransverse position. A fetal blood sample is performed and the pH is reported as 7.2 with a base excess of –7.5 mEq/L.
158. A multiparous woman (previous Cs x1) is having a trial of vaginal delivery after a CS. She progresses to fill dilatation and has been fully for the past 1 hour. She has an epidural and the fetal heart rate is normal. She reports that she is beginning to feel urges to push.

159. A grand multiparous mother had a normal vaginal delivery with an intact perineum about 30 minutes ago. The placenta was delivered by controlled cord traction. She started bleeding and has had syntocinon IM and IV with good uterine contractions but the bleeding is continuing.

160. A primigravida was induced at 38 weeks on account of preeclampsia. She had an ARM and was commenced on syntocinon. She was 3 cm dilated. She has just been examined and the cervix is now 5 cm dilated.

ABNORMAL LABOR

Option list for questions 161–165

A	Amniotic fluid embolism	H	Uterine inversion
B	Cervical tear	I	Uterine rupture
C	Couvelaire uterus	J	
D	Disseminated intravascular coagulation (DIC)	K	
E	Trauma (vaginal or cervical)	L	
F	Thrombocytopenia	M	
G	Uterine atony	N	

Instructions: These women have PPH. Choose from the option list above the most likely cause of the hemorrhage. Each option may be chosen once, more than once, or not at all.

161. A multigravida had a delayed second stage and delivery was expedited with a Wrigley's forceps without an episiotomy. Following delivery, she started hemorrhaging even before the placenta was delivered. The placenta has been delivered and the uterus is well contracted.

162. A multigravida who went into spontaneous labor progressed to 8 cm and then slowed down. Labor was augmented with syntocinon which resulted in regular contractions lasting about 45–60 seconds. About 1 hour after the syntocinon was started she complained of abdominal pains with a bradycardia. When examined she was fully dilated with the head at 0+2. A forceps delivery was performed and she then collapsed after delivery. She is hypotensive and tachycardic with no obvious vaginal bleeding.

163. A primigravida is being induced at 37 weeks for poorly controlled gestational diabetes. The baby is macrosomic and there is polyhydramnios. She was started on syntocinon 6 hours ago. She has developed very sudden chest pain and respiratory distress with associated profound fetal distress. An emergency CS is performed and she is bleeding and the blood is not clotting properly.

164. A 40-year-old multigravida was admitted with abdominal pains at 36 weeks of gestation and absent fetal movements. She had a woody hard uterus on admission and an IUFD confirmed on ultrasound scan. She was induced with syntocinon and progressed very quickly to a normal vaginal delivery with a large retroplacental clot. She is now bleeding and uterotonics have been administered but uterine contractions remain very poor.
165. A multiparous woman has had a normal vaginal delivery and the placenta was delivered by controlled cord traction. There was some difficulty delivering the placenta. Following its delivery, the patient collapses with a BP of 80/40 mm Hg and pulse of 100 bpm. She is bleeding but this is not enough to cause the clinical picture. There is a small dimple on palpation of the uterus.

Option list for questions 166–171

A	ARM and review after 2 hours	**H**	Emergency CS
B	ARM and review after 4 hours	**I**	Fetal blood sample
C	Assisted vaginal delivery	**J**	IV fluids
D	Change position	**K**	IV fluids and paracetamol
E	Commence on syntocinon and review after 2 hours	**L**	SC terbutaline
F	Commence on syntocinon and review after 4 hours	**M**	
G	Correct any dehydration or acidosis/ ketosis	**N**	

Instructions: For each of these women in labor, select from the list of options above the single most appropriate step to take in their management. Each option may be selected once more than once, or not at all.

166. The woman is a primigravida who was admitted in labor at 39 weeks of gestation. The cervix was 5 cm dilated on admission with intact membranes. She has been reassessed and had dilated to 6 cm. She is contracting at a rate of 3–4 in 10 minutes, each contraction lasting about 30–45 seconds.
167. A primigravida had an artificial rupture of fetal membranes 3 hours ago at 6 cm dilatation as labor progress had been slow. She has been contracting at a rate of 3–4 in 10 minutes, each of the contractions lasting for 30–45 seconds. A vaginal examination has just been performed and she if still 6 cm dilated with the vertex at the level of the spines with + molding and + caput.
168. A primigravida with gestational diabetes is being induced at 40 weeks of gestation. She had prostaglandin gel and 8 hours later

started contracting. The cervix then was 5 cm dilated with intact membranes. The CTG over the last 10 minutes is showing variable decelerations with a reduced baseline variability.

169. The woman was admitted in the latent phase of labor 16 hours ago and went into active labor 6 hours ago. She is on Entonox for pain relief. At the last vaginal examination, she was 4 cm dilated with the vertex in the occipitoanterior position at the level of the spines with no molding and no caput. The fetal heart rate now has the following features—an increase in baseline from 150 to 165 bpm, with a normal baseline variability and early decelerations that have been present for the past 30 minutes. Her temperature is 37.6°C.
170. The patient is in the late first state (9 cm) and the fetal heart rate is pathological—there are persistent late decelerations. The liquor draining now is meconium stained and was clear before.
171. The woman is a multigravida in spontaneous labor at 38 weeks of gestation. She has been contracting at the rate of 4–5 in 10 minutes but over the last 10 minutes she is contracting as a rate of 6–7 in 10 minutes, each of the contractions lasting for 30–45 seconds with recurrent late decelerations. The baseline variability has also reduced.

ABNORMAL PRESENTATION

Option list for questions 172–174

A	Allow labor to progress and conduct an assisted breech delivery	H	Fetal blood sample
B	Assisted breech vaginal delivery	I	Fill bladder with saline and proceed to CS
C	Breech extraction	J	Induction of labor
D	Elective CS	K	Operative vaginal delivery
E	Elevate foot of bed	L	
F	Emergency CS	M	
G	ECV and breech extraction	N	

Instructions: For each of these women with an abnormal presentation, select from the option list above the single most appropriate intervention you will recommend. Each option may be chosen once, more than once, or not at all.

172. A multiparous woman comes to the delivery suite with a history of rupture of fetal membranes about 45 minutes ago. She is examined and her vital signs are normal. A CTG shows fetal bradycardia with late and prolonged decelerations. On speculum examination, there is a cord in the vagina and the cervix is 8 cm dilated.

173. A multiparous woman who has had three previous normal vaginal deliveries (birth weights 3.4 kg, 3.6 kg, and 4.0 kg) is admitted in labor at 38 weeks of gestation. The EFW is 3.0 kg. She is examined and found to be 9 cm dilated with a frank breech presenting at the spines.
174. A 36-year-old parous woman with a breech presentation has been assessed, counseled and allowed to have a vaginal breech delivery. She presents in labor at 39 weeks of gestation having ruptured membranes at home. She is examined and the breech which is frank is at the spines in the left sacrotransverse position. An hour after admission, there are persistent variable decelerations and a baseline heart rate that had risen from 144 to 160 pmb.
175. A primigravida is admitted in labor at 40 weeks of gestation. The presenting part is cephalic and is three-fifths palpable per abdomen. Vital signs are stable. At digital examination, the cord is felt behind fetal membranes. A transvaginal ultrasound confirms the diagnosis of cord presentation.

OPERATIVE VAGINAL DELIVERY

Option list for questions 176–178

A	CS category 1	H	Rotation (Kielland) forceps delivery
B	CS category 2	I	Ventouse
C	CS category 3	J	
D	CS category 4	K	
E	Lift out (Wrigley) forceps delivery	L	
F	Manual rotation and forceps delivery	M	
G	Mid-cavity (Neville Barnes) forceps delivery	N	

Instructions: These pregnant women require delivery. For each one, select the best approach to delivery from the option list above. Each option may be chosen once, more than once, or not at all.

176. A primigravida is admitted at 36 weeks with a BP of 150/100 mm Hg and 3+ proteinuria. Bloods have been obtained for preeclampsia investigations and she was placed on an electronic fetal monitor. Over the last 20 minutes, she has been complaining of abdominal pains and the fetal heart shows broad and long-lasting decelerations and reduced baseline variability.
177. A primigravida is admitted with irregular uterine contractions at 39 weeks of gestation. The pregnancy has been uncomplicated and when she last visited the baby was breech. She was scheduled for an

elective CS at 39^{+3} weeks. When examined, she is clinically stable. The cervix is posterior, soft, and the os is closed. She has been placed on a CTG which is showing regular contractions at a frequency of 2–3 in 10 minutes, each lasting 30–45 seconds.

178. A multiparous woman is in labor at 39 weeks of gestation. She progresses to full dilatation and after an hour starts to push. She has been pushing for the past 45 minutes and is now very tired. There is now a fetal bradycardia down to 80 bpm that is not recovering. The head is sitting on the perineum.

EPISIOTOMY AND PERINEAL TEARS

Option list for questions 179–182

A	Cervical tear	**H**	Third-degree perineal tear—IIIB
B	First-degree perineal tear	**I**	Third-degree perineal tear—IIIC
C	Fourth-degree perineal tear	**J**	Vaginal tear
D	Periurethral tear	**K**	
E	Rectovaginal fistula	**L**	
F	Second-degree perineal tear	**M**	
G	Third-degree perineal tear—IIIA	**N**	

Instructions: The women below all had vaginal deliveries with or without assistance and sustained injury to the pelvic floor. For each woman choose from the option list above the type of injury sustained. Each option may be chosen once more than once, or not at all.

179. The woman is a primigravida who had a ventouse delivery because of delayed second stage. She was given an episiotomy with the delivery. The tear has extended to involve the external and internal anal sphincters but not the anal mucosa.
180. The woman had a precipitate labor at term and is now bleeding. The perineum is intact and the uterus is well contracted. The vagina appears intact on palpation.
181. A 30-year-old G2P0, was induced and progressed to full dilatation but developed shoulder dystocia which was managed by the McRoberts maneuver. She sustained a perineal tear which is described as involving >50% of the external anal sphincter but not the rectal mucosa.
182. Following a difficult vaginal delivery, a primigravida develops primary PPH. She has an intact perineum and the uterus is well contracted. During the delivery, the midwife had made several attempts to ease the head out by repeatedly inserting her fingers into an edematous vagina. There is no obvious tear at the vestibule.

POSTPARTUM HEMORRHAGE

Option list for questions 183–187

A	Bilateral internal artery ligation	K	Interventional radiography (uterine artery embolization)
B	Brace suture	L	Intrauterine balloon tamponade (Bakri Balloon)
C	Call for help	M	IV line and cross match at least 4 units of blood
D	Carboprost 0.25 μg intramuscular (IM) every 15 minutes up to eight doses	N	Misoprostol 800 μg sublingual
E	Carboprost intramyometrial 0.5 μg	O	Pack the vagina
F	Coagulation screen including fibrinogen	P	Rub uterine contractions
G	Empty the bladder	Q	Tranexamic acid 1 g intravenously
H	Ergometrine (0.5 mg) slowly intravenously or intramuscularly	R	Syntocinon 40 IU in 100 mL of normal saline intravenously over 4 hours
I	Examination under anesthesia	S	Syntometrine 0.5 IU (500 μg ergometrine and 5 IU syntocinon) intramuscularly or intravenously as a bolus
J	Hysterectomy	T	

Instructions: These women have developed the complication of PPH. For each woman, choose the most appropriate next step in their management. Each option may be chosen once, more than once, or not at all.

183. The woman is a multiparous mother of 4 who has had a normal vaginal delivery. The placenta has just been delivered and the midwife has examined the perineum and it is intact. She also examined the placenta and describes it as complete. A few minutes after delivering the placenta, the woman started bleeding. She has now bled in total about 500 mL. Her bladder had just been emptied prior to delivery.
184. A woman in her second pregnancy delivered with an intact perineum. Following delivery of the placenta she starts bleeding. The uterus is well contracted.
185. The woman is a primigravida who labored for 16 hours and then had an assisted vaginal delivery with a ventouse. Following delivery of the placenta, she started hemorrhaging. Although she has an episiotomy, the bleeding is not coming from it. The uterus is contracting poorly. She has been given various uterotonics and is now on an IV infusion of syntocinon but the bleeding is continuing. Rectal misoprostol 1,000 μg has been given but the bleeding is persisting.

186. A 30-year-old who was induced for gestational diabetes has had a spontaneous vaginal delivery with a left mediolateral episiotomy. IM syntocinon was given with the delivery of the anterior shoulder of the baby. The placenta was delivered by controlled cord traction after 30 minutes. She developed a PPH and was given uterotonics and IV syntocinon (she is still on this). As the bleeding was continuing rectal misoprostol followed by IM carboprost were given. She has been given the eighth dose of carboprost but the bleeding is continuing. After each of the uterotonics the uterus contracts but then relaxes again.

187. The woman is a multipara who delivered spontaneously about 45 minutes ago. The placenta was also delivered spontaneously. She developed PPH which has so far been managed with uterotonics, rectal misoprostol, IM carboprost, and lately a Bakri Balloon. She has continued to bleed and the anesthetists are now anxious about difficulties stabilizing the woman.

Option list for questions 188–191

A	Abnormal coagulation	H	Trauma to the genital tract
B	Amniotic fluid embolism	I	Uterine atony
C	Endometritis	J	Uterine inversion
D	Full bladder	K	Uterine rupture
E	Placental abruption	L	
F	Retained membranes	M	
G	Retained placenta	N	

Instructions: For each of these women with PPH choose from the list of options above the single most likely cause of the hemorrhage. Each option may be chosen once, more than once, or not at all.

188. A woman delivered a few hours ago and the placenta was complete but the membranes were said to be ragged. She is now bleeding from an atonic uterus. Rubbing of the uterus results in contractions that stem the bleeding but once this is stopped the bleeding continues.

189. A primigravida delivered in the pool and was discharged home 6 hours after delivery. The placenta and membrane were complete. Her community midwife has referred her with bleeding 3 days after delivery. She also complains of a brownish vagina discharge and lower abdominal pains but no fever. The uterus is about 14 weeks in size on palpation.

190. A multiparous woman who developed gestational diabetes was induced at 37 weeks because of poor diabetic control. The baby was 4 kg and there was polyhydramnios. She labored for 10 hours and

had a normal vaginal delivery with an intact perineum. The placenta and membranes were complete. Shortly after delivery, she started bleeding briskly.

191. This is a 23-year-old who went into labor spontaneously at 41^{+5} weeks. She progressed to full cervical dilatation and had a normal vaginal delivery with an episiotomy. The third stage was managed with IM syntocinon. Following delivery of the placenta she started bleeding. Her uterus is well contracted.

Option list for questions 192–196

A	Cervical, vaginal, and/or perineal tears	**H**	Placenta previa
B	Chorioamnionitis (infection)	**I**	Polyhydramnios
C	Fetal macrosomia	**J**	PPH
D	Induction of labor	**K**	Prolonged labor with or without augmentation
E	Instrumental delivery	**L**	Syntocinon augmentation
F	Maternal obesity	**M**	Uterine fibroids
G	Multiple pregnancy	**N**	

Instructions: The following women all developed PPH after delivery. Choose from the option list above the most likely risk factor from each woman's history that is most likely associated with the hemorrhage. Each option may be selected once, more than once, or not at all.

192. A 38-year-old who had IVF that resulted in twin pregnancies delivered after a 12-hour labor at 38 weeks of gestation. She is now bleeding and has lost in total 700 mL of blood.
193. The woman is 28 years old in her first pregnancy. When she booked for antenatal care, her BMI was 38 kg/m^2. She went into spontaneous labor at 39 weeks and delivered after 12 hours in the first stage. Following delivery of the placenta she started bleeding. She was given an episiotomy but the bleeding is not from the episiotomy.
194. A 24-year-old primigravida was induced at 38 weeks because of preeclampsia. 8 hours after she had 12 mg of Propess® (dinoprostone) vaginally, she started contracting regularly. A few hours later she had spontaneous rupture of fetal membranes when the cervix was 4 cm. 4 hours later she was still 4 cm and therefore labor was augmented with syntocinon. 8 hours later she had progressed to full cervical dilation and after 2 hours in the second stage, had a normal vaginal delivery. The third stage was managed actively with syntocinon. She has developed primary PPH.
195. This woman, a primigravida was admitted in labor at 39 weeks. Her cervix was 3 cm dilated and she had ruptured fetal membranes.

At the time of admission, she was having 3–4 contractions every 10 minutes, each lasting between 30 and 45 seconds. 4 hours later she had dilated to 4 cm and when reassessed after 4 hours had dilated to 5 cm. Syntocinon was therefore commenced and she progressed to full dilatation after 14 hours. She then remained in the passive second stage for 2 hours and thereafter pushed for 1 hour before having a ventouse delivery because of maternal exhaustion.

196. This woman was induced for prolonged prelabor rupture of membranes. She originally presented with ruptured membranes at 32 weeks of gestation and was managed expectantly. She was induced is at 36 weeks of gestation on account of a rising maternal pulse, fetal tachycardia, and C-reactive protein (CRP). She had a normal vaginal delivery and started bleeding. The uterus has remained poorly contracted. The induction-to-delivery interval was 10 hours.

PUERPERIUM AND PUERPERAL DISORDERS

Option list for questions 197–200

A	Breast abscess	H	Pulmonary embolism
B	Bronchopneumonia	I	Tonsillitis
C	DVT—pelvic	J	Urinary tract infections (pyelonephritis)
D	Endometritis	K	Wound infection
E	Lobar pneumonia	L	
F	Mastitis	M	
G	Meningitis	N	

Instructions: For each of these women with a diagnosis of puerperal pyrexia, choose from the list of options above the single most likely cause of the pyrexia. Each option may be chosen once, more than once, or not at all.

197. This is a woman who delivered 3 days ago and now presents with fever chills, painful micturition, and lower abdominal pains. She has a reddish vaginal discharge. On examination she has a temperature of 38.3°C, a pulse of 98 beats/min (bpm) and a BP of 130/73 mm Hg. The uterus is about 14 weeks but is not tender. There is mild tenderness on the sides of the abdomen. A urinalysis shows +++ red blood cells, ++ leukocytes, and ++ nitrites.

198. Four days after an emergency CS, a woman is admitted with a temperature of 38.5°C, chest pain, and cough which is productive of rusty sputum. On examination she is pyrexial (temperature 38.5°C), tachycardic (pulse =108 bpm), and normotensive (BP = 110/65 mm Hg). There is dullness on percussion as well as bronchial breath sounds on the right lower lung lobe anteriorly and posteriorly. Her uterus has

involuted to 12 weeks and there is mild tenderness over the wound which is mildly reddish.

199. A week after a normal vaginal delivery a 39-year-old grand multiparous women presents with chest pains and difficulties breathing of sudden onset. She is examined and found to be pyrexial (temperature = 38.0°C), tachycardic (pulse = 110 bpm) and hypertensive (BP =140/90 mm Hg). Her oxygen saturations in air vary between 90 and 94%. There are no crepitations or bronchial breath sounds on auscultation of the chest. Her uterus is well involuted.

200. Five days after delivery a mother is admitted feeling unwell and feverish. She complaints of buttocks pains and swollen feet. Although her feet were swollen in pregnancy, these have got worse and are now mildly painful. She has no cough and is breastfeeding with no problems. When examined she is pyrexial (temperature = 37.9°C), tachycardic (pulse = 105 bpm) and normotensive (BP = 135/83 mm Hg). There are no abnormal features on chest examination. The uterus is well involuted and not tender. There is bilateral edema of the lower limbs extending up the mid-thigh. Although the right is more than the left and slightly warmer there is no tenderness and Homan's sign is negative.

LACTATION

Option list for questions 201 and 202

A	Bloods stained discharge	H	Mastitis
B	Breast abscess	I	Painful nipples
C	Breast cancer	J	Retracted nipple
D	Breast engorgement	K	
E	Breast lump	L	
F	Cracked nipple	M	
G	Fibroma	N	

Instructions: Choose from the option list above the single most likely diagnosis in each of the women presenting with breast symptoms post-partum. Each option may be selected once, more than once, or not at all.

201. The woman is a primigravida who saw her community midwife 2 days after delivery complaining that the baby is struggling to latch onto the breast and as such is crying all the time. The breasts are engorged but not inflamed and nipples are not prominent on inspection.

202. On the fifth day postpartum a primigravida attends the emergency with flu-like symptoms, fever, and rigors. She is breastfeeding but says that her daughter has not been able to feed from the left breast. This is found on examination to be engorged, red and warm to touch.

PERINATAL AND MATERNAL MORTALITY

Option list for questions 203–206

A	Direct maternal mortality	H	Neonatal mortality rate
B	Early neonatal death	I	Perinatal mortality
C	Fortuitous maternal death	J	Perinatal mortality rate
D	Indirect maternal mortality	K	Stillbirth
E	Infant death	L	Stillbirth rate
F	Late neonatal death	M	
G	Neonatal mortality	N	

Instructions: For each of the descriptions below, choose from the list of options above the single most appropriate nomenclature. Each option may be chosen once, more than once, or not at all.

203. Death occurring as a result of pregnancy or its complications.
204. Death of the mother from conditions which might be made worse in pregnancy.
205. A newborn at 21 weeks of gestation who had only a heartbeat at birth and was not resuscitated.
206. Death of a woman at 30 weeks of gestation with pancreatic cancer that developed during pregnancy.

FEMALE GENITAL MUTILATION

Option list for questions 207–209

A	Active management of third stage with or without syntocinon infusion	H	Group and save
B	Deinfibulation around 20 weeks	I	Infibulation
C	Deinfibulation at the time of delivery	J	Intravenous (IV) access
D	Deinfibulation intrapartum	K	Post-traumatic stress disorder (PTSD)
E	Deinfibulation postdelivery	L	Referral for psychological/psychiatric assessment
F	Epidural	M	Screen for blood borne infections (HIV and hepatitis B and C)
G	Episiotomy with delivery	N	

Instructions: These women are either attending for antenatal assessment or to book for antenatal care or in labor. Each woman gives a history of female genital mutilation (FGM). For each woman, choose the most appropriate management plan from the list of options above. Each option may be chosen once, more than once, or not at all.

207. A 25-year-old is attending for her first pregnancy. She gives a history of circumcision when she was 8 years old. She arrived in the country

3 years ago to join her husband. She says that sexual intercourse has been very painful. She is examined and the clitoris is absent. There is mild scarring at the introitus but it is able to admit two fingers. She has just had all the bloods for investigations including HIV and hepatitis B and C.

208. A 28-year-old primigravida is now 12 weeks. She booked for antenatal care at 10 weeks and has had various investigations. She was referred to the psychologist for assessment after her booking visit. At that visit, the introitus was examined and found to be very narrow and could only admit one finger. She is otherwise well and her NT scan today was normal. She has had a blood test for the combined aneuploidy test.

209. A 23-year-old with FGM type 3 was admitted in labor at 40 weeks of gestation. She had had a deinfibulation at 20 weeks. The pregnancy was uncomplicated. She was examined on admission with some difficulties and the cervix was 6 cm dilated. An epidural was recommended and inserted. She is now ready to start pushing.

APPLIED GENETICS IN OBSTETRICS AND GYNECOLOGY

Option list for questions 210–213

A	Autosomal dominant inheritance	H	Mosaicism
B	Autosomal recessive inheritance	I	Multifactorial inheritance
C	Deletion	J	Mutation
D	Duplication	K	Polygenic inheritance
E	Inversion	L	Sex-linked autosomal recessive inheritance
F	Imprinting inheritance	M	Translocation
G	Mitochondrial inheritance	N	

Instructions: For each of these cases, choose from the option list above the single best mode of inheritance. Each option may be selected once, more than once, or not at all.

210. The parents have been seen for prepregnancy counseling. One of them has a condition in the heterozygous form but manifests the condition while the other is unaffected. Following counseling they are told that they will produce a 1:1 ratio of affected to unaffected offspring.

211. The woman is 8 weeks into their first pregnancy and her Hb genotype is HbAS while that of her partner is HbAC. They have been told that

their offspring have a 1:4 chance of having sickle cell disease (SCD) and a 2:4 chance of being carriers.

212. The woman is 30 years and this is her first pregnancy. She indicates that her brother suffers from a bleeding disorder for which she is a carrier. Her husband is normal. They have been told that the condition she has expresses itself more in males than females and that they have a 50% of having affected sons and 50% chance of having carrier daughters.

213. A woman had a high-risk aneuploidy test at 12 weeks and was offered CVS. The result has come back as 45XO/46XX.

Part C: Answer and Explanations

1. **(K) Second trimester.** Pregnancy is divided into trimesters—the first trimester is the period from conception to 13/14 weeks, the second trimester is from 13/14 weeks to 28 weeks and the third trimester is from 29 to 42 weeks.
2. **(A) Bartholomew's rule.** Abdominal palpation allows for clinical assessment of the size of the pregnancy and its relationship to the gestational age. Bartholomew's rule equates specific anatomical landmarks on the abdomen to specific gestational ages. This is the basis for symphysiofundal height measurements (SFM).
3. **(D) Leopold's maneuvers.** An obstetric examination aims to determine the size of the pregnancy (fundal height) the lie of the baby (longitudinal, transverse, or oblique) and presentation including the attitude and the position of the fetus. The maneuvers used for this were first described by Leopold.
4. **(I) Parity.** Parity and gravidity are terms used to designate the total number of previous pregnancies that progressed beyond viability (24 weeks) irrespective or outcome and the total number of pregnancies (current and previous) irrespective of the outcomes (i.e., including miscarriages and ectopic), respectively.
5. **(C) Anomaly ultrasound scan.** At 18 weeks, the only investigation that would be ordered apart from a urinalysis which she has already had is a detailed ultrasound scan (anomaly ultrasound scan). This is performed between 18 and 20 weeks. No other blood tests are routinely collected unless clinically indicated at this stage.
6. **(H) Glucose tolerance test.** This woman has two risk factors for gestational diabetes—her weight (she is obese) and a previous macrosomic baby (4.5 kg). The test to order at this stage is an oral glucose tolerance test (OGTT) which is performed at 24–28 weeks
7. **(N) Urine microscopy, culture, and sensitivity.** There are no routine investigations that have to be performed at 16 weeks unless clinically indicated. The presence of nitrites, leukocytes, and protein in urine is highly suggestive of a urinary tract infection although the patient is asymptomatic. Urine culture is the most appropriate investigation at this stage.
8. **(K) Routine booking investigations.** Having had her dating ultrasound scan which has been described as normal it can be assumed that the NT was measured and was normal. What is required now are the routine booking blood investigations. These are not normally done before 10 weeks hence they would not have been done at 9 weeks.

9. **(A) BP.** BP falls to a nadir in the second trimester and then rises back to prepregnancy levels by the beginning of the third trimester.
10. **(G) Platelet count.** During pregnancy, platelet count falls but reactivity increases especially in the second and third trimesters. This then falls to normal levels by 12 weeks of postpartum.
11. **(C) Cardiac output.** Cardiac output increases by about 40%; in most women this translates to an increase from 4.5 L/min to 6.0 L/min but there is a further increase of about 2 L/min in labor.
12. **(C) Constitutional.** The patient is underweight and her pregnancy has been uncomplicated. The most likely cause of the small baby she has is constitutional rather than pathological.
13. **(H) High BMI—maternal obesity.** The baby is macrosomic. With regards to risk factors on the list of options the two possibilities are type II diabetes and maternal obesity. As the pregnancy has been uncomplicated, the most likely risk factor associated with the fetal macrosomia is maternal obesity. If polyhydramnios had been associated with the macrosomia, diabetes would be a risk factor.
14. **(D) Duodenal atresia.** Causes of polyhydramnios include diabetes, fetal infections, and congenital malformations that affect swallowing or passage of fluid through the gastrointestinal tract. As this has been an uncomplicated pregnancy, diabetes is unlikely and furthermore the fetus is not macrosomic. The only other possible cause of the polyhydramnios is a structural abnormality and in this case duodenal atresia which is more common in male fetuses is most likely.
15. **(B) Chronic renal disease.** This fetus has early-onset fetal growth restriction (as evidenced by AC and HC below the 10th centile and reduced liquor volume). The most likely cause of this is a chronic maternal disease like chronic renal disease.
16. **(J) Stillbirth rate.**
17. **(G) Perinatal mortality rate.**
18. **(H) Neonatal death rate.**
19. **(A) Early direct maternal mortality.**
20. **(E) Late indirect maternal mortality.**
21. **(C) Continue SFM antenatally.** This is a low-risk pregnancy and there is no need to order any additional test for the women or for the baby. She should therefore continue with her routine antenatal care with the measurement of the symphysiofundal height.
22. **(I) Ultrasound for fetal growth.** One of the most important factors for fetal growth restriction is previous fetal growth restriction. This is an indication for serial growth scans as clinical palpation is not sensitive enough to identify most growth restricted babies.

23. **(F) NIPD.** It is now possible to determine the Hb genotype of the baby from circulating free fetal DNA in maternal circulation by means of a noninvasive prenatal diagnostic test at 10–12 weeks. This is accurate and associated with no complications. While CVS and amniocentesis will also allow for determination of the Hb genotype of the fetus they both carry the risk of miscarriage and the procedures are invasive.
24. **(G) NIPT.** Noninvasive prenatal testing although a screening rest will provide a risk estimate of >99% for trisomies 12, 18, and 21. These are the most common aneuploidies compatible with live and if the risk for these are low she could be counseled about the possibilities of other aneuploidies and referred for a cardiac echo at 22–24 weeks.
25. **(K) Refer for anomaly scan and cardiac echo at 22–24 weeks.** Although the NT is raised in this patient, the combined screening test (i.e., NT and biochemistry) has classified her as low risk. She should therefore be referred for a routine anomaly ultrasound scan and a fetal echo at 22–24 weeks as isolated high NT's are associated with a higher risk of cardiac and other structural malformations.
26. **(G) NIPT.** At 15 weeks, she cannot be offered the combined NT and biochemistry test as this is done between 11 and 13^{+6} weeks. Furthermore, an invasive test in the form of amniocentesis, while being able to establish whether her baby has aneuploidy or not, is associated with a risk of miscarriage and therefore the best option would be a screening test with the quadruple test. An NIPT would be ideal as it will provide a high detection rate for aneuploidy (higher than that for the quadruple test) without risking the pregnancy.
27. **(H) Spina bifida.** Open spina bifida is characterized by a lemon-shaped skull and a banana-shaped cerebellum. The presence of these abnormalities is pathognomonic of open spina bifida. Ultrasound should diagnose >95% of these abnormalities antenatally.
28. **(F) Exomphalos.** There are two types of anterior abdominal wall defects—gastroschisis and exomphalos. In the latter, there is a membrane covering the bowel with the cord inserted at the apex of the membrane. It is associated with an increased risk of aneuploidy especially trisomy 18 and facial defects. Karyotyping is therefore indicated in this patient.
29. **(D) Diaphragmatic hernia.** Diaphragmatic hernia is a congenital malformations whose diagnosis can be missed if later ultrasound scans are not routinely performed. This is because some of these are not obvious with early ultrasound scans. The diagnosis is based on the present of intra-abdominal structures (stomach most commonly, but also the liver and bowel) in the chest with associated mediastinal shift. Later in pregnancy, there may be an associated polyhydramnios.

30. **(G) Gastroschisis.** There are two types of anterior abdominal wall defects—gastroschisis and exomphalos. In the former, there is no membrane covering the bowel which floats freely in the amniotic cavity with the cord inserting laterally to the defect. This abnormality is not associated with chromosomal abnormalities although preterm delivery is common. It is also not an indication for CS.
31. **(B) Normal discordant twin growth.** In this patient, the scans show an estimated weight difference of 150 g between the fetuses with normal liquor volume and Dopplers. This is an expected weight difference in twin pregnancies. Selective growth restriction is defined as weight differences of >20% and in this case the difference is <15%. There are no other abnormalities (liquor volume and Dopplers are all normal).
32. **(G) Stage II TTTS.** TTTS is classified into four stages (Quintero stages I to IV) based on the Doppler abnormalities combined with oligohydramnios/polyhydramnios sequence and the presence of absence of the bladder. In this case, the bladder is not seen in the smaller (donor twin) but the Dopplers are normal and these are features of Stage II. When Dopplers are abnormal it is stage III, when there is hydrops in one but both are alive it is stage IV and when one of the fetuses is dead that is stage V.
33. **(C) Selective fetal growth restriction.** The definition of selective fetal growth restriction in twin pregnancies is where the estimated weight difference is >20% with or without abnormal Dopplers. In this patient, there is >20% estimated weight difference and when the Dopplers are normal, this is considered stage I.
34. **(A) Cord entanglement.** The most common complication of MC monoamniotic twin pregnancy is cord entanglement which is said to occur in nearly all the pregnancies. The increased activity of the twins most likely resulted in cord entanglement and the slowing of their movements reflects the degree of strangulation in the cord. A delay delivery in this case is likely to result in intrauterine fetal death (IUFD).
35. **(F) Elective CS at 32–34 weeks.** This patient has MC monoamniotic twins and the greatest risk of this type of twins is cord entanglement and sudden IUFD of one or both twins. It is therefore strongly recommended that once that twins reach 32 weeks delivery should be considered and this must be by CS.
36. **(E) Corticosteroids and delivery by CS.** TTTS is best treated by laser division of the chorionic plate but this should be mainly up to 28–30 weeks. In this patient, the pregnancy is already past 32 weeks and the babies are best delivered and the anemia/polycythemia managed postnatally rather than exposing them to the risk of laser therapy.

37. **(K) Induction of labor at 37–38 weeks.** The recommended timing of delivery is 37–38 weeks for uncomplicated twins. Where the first twin is cephalic and there are no contraindications, the aim should be for a vaginal delivery hence the recommendation is induction of labor at 37–38 weeks.
38. **(H) Elective CS at 37–38 weeks.** The recommended timing of delivery is 37–38 weeks for uncomplicated twins. Where the first twin is cephalic and there are no contraindications, the aim should be for a vaginal delivery, however, when the presentation of the first twin is abnormal (as in this patient) then an elective CS is recommended at 37–38 weeks.
39. **(F) Placental abruption.** The two major causes of antepartum hemorrhage are placental previa and abruption. The former presents with painless bleeding while the latter presents with painful bleeding and an irritable uterus. Her age is a risk factor for placental abruption.
40. **(D) Heavy show.** This woman has had two preterm deliveries which means she is more likely to have another preterm birth. She now presents with vaginal bleeding associated with intermittent lower abdominal pains which radiate to the back (characteristic of uterine contractions). Any vaginal bleeding mixed with mucous is more likely to be a heavy show especially when this occurs at the time of possible labor.
41. **(J) Placenta percreta.** Previous CS is a risk factor for placenta previa. In this patient, the placenta is, however, not previa but appears to be penetrating into the myometrium hence it is a percreta placenta. It is not unusual for this to be part of placenta previa especially in those who have had a CS as in this patient.
42. **(F) Low-lying placenta.** Placentas are either low lying, previa or normally sited on ultrasound scan. A normally sited placenta is >2 cm from the internal os while placentals that cover the internal os are previa and those that are <2 cm from the internal os as described as low lying. Most of the low-lying placentas by the time delivery would become normally sited (so-called placental migration).
43. **(B) CS at 34–36 weeks.** Following the diagnosis of vasa previa, delivery must be planned for 34–36 weeks to avoid the risk of rupture with onset of spontaneous labor. Such a patient may have to be admitted to the hospital until delivery.
44. **(H) Transvaginal ultrasound scan.** There is needed to exclude or confirm a low lying or placenta previa in this patient and the best approach is a transvaginal ultrasound scan.
45. **(A) Admit from 28 weeks.** This patient has placenta previa that has already presented with bleeding albeit this was mild. She should be admitted at 28 weeks and managed as inpatient until delivery by CS at 37–38 weeks or earlier if she goes into labor.

46. **(C) Eclampsia.** Eclampsia is the occurrence of seizures in a patient with preeclampsia. This can occur antenatally, intrapartum, or postpartum. The occurrent of eclampsia is an indication for delivery and commencement of intravenous (IV) magnesium sulfate.
47. **(I) Pregnancy-induced (gestational) hypertension.** When hypertension occurs for the first time in the second half of pregnancy without any other complications such as hematological/biochemical derangement and no proteinuria it is considered gestational or pregnancy-induced hypertension. This may progress to preeclampsia or remain as hypertension.
48. **(D) Essential hypertension.** This patient is hypertensive in the first trimester with no other associated factors to explain the hypertension. The most likely diagnosis is essential hypertension as most of these are asymptomatic and diagnosed incidentally as in this patient. She is, however, at risk of preeclampsia.
49. **(F) HELLP syndrome.** When preeclampsia is complicated by low platelets and elevated liver enzymes as in this patient the diagnosis is HELLP syndrome (hypertension low platelets and elevated liver enzymes).
50. **(E) Labetalol.** This patient needs treatment for her hypertension as although she is minimally symptomatic, she could suffer from intracranial hemorrhage. The treatment of choice would be labetalol which should be given orally in the first instance.
51. **(F) IV magnesium sulfate.** This patient has severe preeclampsia which is an indication for initiating IV magnesium sulfate. Although her BP is not at a level that requires urgent treatment, her symptoms suggest that she would develop eclampsia if not placed on magnesium sulfate. This will also help lower the BP although starting her on antihypertensives would be the next stage in her management.
52. **(F) IV magnesium sulfate.** The treatment of choice for eclampsia is IV magnesium sulfate. The dose is 4 g IV start over 10–15 minutes followed by 1 g/h maintenance dose.
53. **(B) Emergency CS.** Any woman who is started on magnesium sulfate to control fits to prevent progression to eclampsia should be delivered once she is stable. The mode of delivery should be determined by the state of the cervix. If this is favorable a vaginal delivery is preferred. In this patient, the cervix is unfavorable and induction of labor will be prolonged and likely to predispose to fits hence the best approach to her management.
54. **(D) Ultrasound sound for fetal growth and umbilical artery Doppler.** This patient is hypertensive as well and also had abnormal uterine artery Dopplers at 20 weeks, hence at risk of having a growth restricted

fetus and preeclampsia. She should therefore be having serial growth ultrasound scans as well as umbilical artery Dopplers every 4–6 weeks.

55. **(I) Urine spot PCR.** When significant proteinuria is identified, the proteinuria should be quantified by a spot PCR or 24-hour urine protein estimation. Spot PCR would be the first approach in this patient followed by routine bloods for preeclampsia.
56. **(G) Urinalysis.** Any patient who attends the antenatal clinic should have her urine checked for protein leukocytes and glucose. This is more so when she is hypertensive. This patient has two risk factors for preeclampsia— (1) her age and (2) parity. It is therefore important to check for proteinuria.
57. **(D) Commence on folic acid 5 mg daily.** This woman has had renal and retinal assessments in the last 3 months and her HbA1C is indicative of good diabetic control. She can therefore start trying for a baby but should be placed on folic acid 5 mg daily and advised to continue with this until the 12 weeks of gestation.
58. **(G) Measure HbA1C and commence on folic acid.** This patient had a renal and retinal assessment <3 months previously hence does not need another one. However, there is no information about her latest HbA1C so this should be measured and she should be commenced on folic acid 5 mg. If the HbA1C is <10 she can start trying, although ideally this should be around 6.5%.
59. **(I) Renal and retinal assessment.** This patient has a relatively well-controlled diabetes and can therefore embark on pregnancy. However, it would be useful to assess her eyes and kidney function since she last had some form of assessment 6 months previously. Additionally, she should be commenced on folic acid 5 mg daily.
60. **(C) Change antihypertensives and commence on contraception and folic acid.** This patient is on an ACE inhibitor which is not advisable in pregnancy as it is teratogenic. She should therefore switch this to a less teratogenic option and her BP well controlled before she becomes pregnant. She should therefore be given an effective contraceptive and commenced on folic acid 5 mg daily.
61. **(L) Start on metformin.** This patient's blood glucose levels are demonstrating poor control with diet and in the first instance she should be commenced on metformin and if this fails to control her diabetes, she would be started on insulin.
62. **(K) Start on insulin.** The indications for starting women with diabetes diagnosed in pregnancy on insulin include poor control as evidence by high blood glucose levels on metformin and complications that reflect poor control such as polyhydramnios and fetal macrosomia (as in this patient). The normal blood glucose values in the 2 days

before consultation are not unusual as patients would religiously ensure that these values are normal prior to clinic visits.

63. **(C) Fasting blood glucose at 6-13 weeks.** This woman who was diagnosed with gestational diabetes mellitus (GDM) and has delivered should be screened for type II diabetes at 6–13 weeks with a fasting blood glucose. She has an increased risk of developing type II diabetes and should also have annual screening for diabetes.
64. **(I) Glucose tolerance test at 24–28 weeks.** Indications for OGTT at 24–28 weeks include obesity, previous macrosomic babies, family history in first-degree relative, previous macrosomia or unexplained stillbirth, or congenital malformations. This patient has had two previous macrosomic babies and should therefore have an OGTT at 24–28 weeks of gestation.
65. **(J) Revert to prepregnancy dose of metformin.** The placenta is responsible for the diabetogenic effects of pregnancy and following its delivery, the requirements for diabetogenic medications return to prepregnancy levels very quickly. In this patient therefore, the insulin should be stopped and she reverts to prepregnancy metformin levels. For those women who are diagnosed in pregnancy, all agents to control blood glucose levels should be stopped.
66. **(F) Hyperthyroidism.** The clinical features this patient presents with are characteristic of hyperthyroidism. In addition to these features, she may also have pretibial myxedema and exophthalmos.
67. **(G) Hypothyroidism.** Most women with hypothyroidism in pregnancy are asymptomatic. Those with symptoms present with a variety of clinical features which include weight gain, intolerance to cold, constipation fatigue, and somnolence. Examination features include delay or relaxation of the deep tendon reflexes.
68. **(C) Cushing's syndrome.** Cushing's syndrome is a rare endocrine disorder in pregnancy characterized by increased glucocorticoid production (commonly due to excessive ACTH production). The symptoms include weight gain, striae, weakness, glucose intolerance, hypertension, and in some cases features of preeclampsia.
69. **(E) Pemphigoid gestationis.** Pemphigoid gestationis also known as pregnancy-induced bullous pemphigoid or gestational pemphigoid or herpes gestationis characteristically presents in the second half of pregnancy with a rash that is typically around the umbilicus and then spreads to the trunk, extremities, and palms and soles but not involving the mucosa. The rash starts as an urticaria that then fuse to form clusters of blisters (bullae) which on clinical examination appear as large and tense blisters mainly around the edges of the rash.
70. **(F) Polymorphic eruption of pregnancy (PEP).** Polymorphic eruption of pregnancy also known as pruritic urticarial papules or plaques

of pregnancy or toxic erythema of pregnancy present in the third trimester or immediately postpartum with itching and a rash that characteristically spares the periumbilical area. The rash starts on the abdomen and spreads to involve the trunk and extremities but rarely affects the palms and soles.

71. **(B) Atopic eruption of pregnancy.** Atopic eruptions of pregnancy (also known as eczema of pregnancy or prurigo gestationis or nurses early-onset prurigo of pregnancy) is characterized by an itching rash that develops around 25–30 weeks. The rash which is typically found on the face, trunk, and extensor surfaces of the limbs is erythematous with excoriations from scratching.
72. **(B) Bronchopneumonia.** The clinical features are in keeping with a chest infection and one where there is widespread pathology. Generalized crackles in the presence of a temperature and systemic symptoms are highly suggestive of bronchopneumonia. A rusty sputum is characteristic of *Haemophilus influenzae* infection.
73. **(F) Lobar pneumonia.** The clinical features in this patient are indicative of consolidation, hence diagnostic of lobar pneumonia. This is often associated with systemic symptoms.
74. **(K) Tension pneumothorax.** Lateralizing signs without systemic symptoms and absence of a temperature suggest a noninfective pathology. This could either be from a collapse lung (in which case the tracheal deviation will be away from the collapsed side) or pneumothorax in which case the deviation will be toward to side with the pneumothorax as in this case.
75. **(D) Chest-X-ray.** An appropriate investigation in this woman is a CXR. These are not contraindicated in pregnancy but it is advisable that the gravid uterus is shielded during the examination. While sputum culture would be an important investigation confirmation of chest pathology by X-ray will allow for initiation of appropriate treatment. The culture and sensitivity will help with antibiotic choice if there is no response to the initial antibiotic treatment.
76. **(B) Bronchial lavage for PCR.** Tuberculosis will have to be confirmed by either sputum culture/PCR or bronchial lavage and PCR from the lavage. Since this patient is not producing any sputum, lavage will have to be performed to obtain a sample for PCR. This is the most accurate diagnostic test for pulmonary tuberculosis.
77. **(H) Pulse oximetry.** This patient presenting with breathing difficulties and possibly cyanosed needs an urgent pulse oximetry as this will determine how much oxygen she should be given by face mask.
78. **(C) Commence on aspirin from 12 weeks until delivery and LMWH until 6 weeks of postpartum.** Systemic lupus erythematosus is associated with several complications in pregnancy including miscarriages,

fetal growth restriction, placental abruption, preeclampsia, venous thromboembolism (VTE), and heart block. Starting aspirin from 12 weeks until delivery combined with LMWH from now until 6 weeks of postpartum has been shown to improve outcome in these women.

79. **(F) Anti-Ro/La antibodies.** This baby has pathology consistent with congenital heart block. This is associated with anti-Ro and La antibodies which should therefore be measured in this patient.
80. **(K) Manage pregnancy as normal.** Rheumatoid arthritis is a chronic autoimmune condition that affects the big joints. About 75% of women will experience improvements in pregnancy but over 90% will have a flare postpartum. It is not known to have an adverse effect on pregnancy hence the pregnancy should be managed as normal.
81. **(G) Elective CS at 38–39 weeks.** It is very difficult to monitor the heart rate of fetuses with congenital heart block in labor hence these women should be delivered electively. If she presents in labor then an emergency CS should be performed.
82. **(E) Marfan syndrome.** Marfan syndrome is a connective tissue disorder that is inherited as an autosomal dominant condition. There is often a valvular disorder—commonly mitral valve prolapse, aortic regurgitation, and dissection. The mortality in these patients is up to 50% especially in those with marked aortic root dissection.
83. **(J) Pulmonary stenosis.** The symptoms of pulmonary stenosis are essentially those of right sided heart failure with chest pressure and pain. This is not a symptom of congestive heart failure.
84. **(H) Myocardial infarction.** Raised troponin levels are pathogno monic of myocardial infarction. This (chest pressure) is more common in the third trimester but can occur in all trimester.
85. **(A) Aortic root dissecting aneurysm.** Aneurysms present with sudden-onset piercing/stabbing pain that radiates to the back. Interscapular pain is characteristic of aortic root dissection.
86. **(D) Delay pregnancy for 6–12 months.** Ideally, she should wait for 12–24 months and only embark on pregnancy when the renal function is normal (proteinuria is <500 mg/ 24 hours) and serum creatinine is <1.5 mg/dL, she is on minimal immunosuppressants (at most 15 mg/ day of prednisolone) and her BP is <140/90 mm Hg.
87. **(F) Renal ultrasound scan.** Recurrent urinary tract infection (especially pyelonephritis is an indication for renal ultrasound scan in pregnancy. Infection with *Pseudomonas species* is an indication for renal ultrasound scan even if it is the first episode as this infection is likely related to malformations of the renal tract or renal calculi.
88. **(G) Screen for GDM by OGTT at 24–28 weeks.** Women who have had transplant are at risk of gestational diabetes and should therefore

be screened for this in pregnancy. This patient has had most of the interventions recommended but needs an OGTT.

89. **(I) Switch ACE inhibitor to a less teratogenic option, start folic acid and give contraception.** This patient is on an ACE inhibitor which is contraindicated in pregnancy. This should be discontinued and a less teratogenic option substituted. It is important that this is allowed to control her BP before she embarks on pregnancy hence she should be given appropriate contraception and also commenced on folic acid 5 mg daily.
90. **(P) *Toxoplasma gondii.*** Toxoplasmosis is an infection caused by the protozoan *Toxoplasma gondii*. It is transmitted through drinking contaminated water or eating meat contaminated with the oocytes. Most infected women are asymptomatic (>95% of cases) and for those with symptoms, these tend to be nonspecific and include flu-like symptoms, myalgia, low-grade pyrexia, and lymphadenopathy. Vertical transmission is associated with congenital malformations which include ventriculomegaly, intracranial, and hepatic calcifications.
91. **(D) CMV.** The CMV is the most common viral infection in pregnancy. Most infected women are asymptomatic. Symptoms are nonspecific and include flu-like illness, malaise, myalgia, fever, and cervical lymphadenopathy. Vertical transmission in the first trimester is associated with various congenital malformations which include fetal growth restriction, microcephaly, hepatosplenomegaly, and calcifications in the brain and liver.
92. **(O) Syphilis.** Infections with the spirochaete *Treponema pallidum* which causes syphilis can be primary, secondary, or tertiary. Primary syphilis is characterized by painless genital ulcers which last for about 3–8 weeks. The ulcers are typically bilateral and often described as kissing.
93. **(Q) Tuberculosis.** Pulmonary tuberculosis presents with cough which may or may not be productive; there may be hemoptysis (coughing up blood) and often the patient will complain of night sweats. Culture of sputum in most cases is negative unless Ziehl–Neelsen staining is performed. The most accurate diagnosis is from PCR of a bronchoalveolar lavage.
94. **(M) Parvovirus B19.** Parvovirus is a common infection amongst children and typically presents with fever a rash and red cheeks (also known as slapped cheek-disease). Its symptoms are nonspecific. It is an important cause of nonimmune hydrops. The diagnosis in this patient is based on her profession and the history of the infection in the children in her class.
95. **(A) Chickenpox.** Chickenpox is an infection which confers lifelong immunity in almost everyone who has had the infection.

It is characterized by a maculopapular rash on trunk and limbs. The diagnosis in this patient is based on her history, her occupation, and the nature of the symptoms. Confirmation of diagnosis will be by serology.

96. **(B) *Chlamydia trachomatis.*** The two causes of sticky neonatal eyes are *Chlamydia trachomatis* and *Neisseria gonorrhoeae*. The onset of symptoms from the former is 5–14 days after birth while the latter is 2–4 days. In this case, the symptoms were of onset 7 days after delivery.
97. **(L) *Neisseria gonorrhoeae.*** The two causes of sticky neonatal eyes are *Chlamydia trachomatis* and *Neisseria gonorrhoeae*. The onset of symptoms from the former is 5–14 days after birth while the latter is 2–4 days. In this case the symptoms were of onset 2 days after delivery.
98. **(K) Malaria.** Malaria is a tropical infection caused by the protozoal *Plasmodium*. It typically presents with fever, chills, muscle aches, and joint paints with associated chills. The fever is characteristic in its pattern—getting worse in the evenings.
99. **(H) HIV.** HIV is an immunodeficiency infection that causes a low CD4+ count and therefore predisposes the individual to opportunistic infections. High-risk groups include homosexuals, IV drug abusers, and individuals from high-risk countries especially those of sub-Sahara Africa.
100. **(C) Coronavirus.** Coronavirus-19 is caused by the coronavirus severe acute respiratory syndrome coronavirus-2 (SARS-CoV-2). Its clinical features include nonproductive cough fever, nasal congestion, nausea, vomiting, diarrhea, myalgia, headaches, and recent loss of smell and taste. Diagnosis is by PCR of flock nasopharyngeal swabs or saliva. CT or plain X-rays of the chest often show characteristic ground glass pneumonia in those with moderate to severe disease. Other features include lymphopenia and raised procalcitonin levels especially in those with superimposed bacterial infections
101. **(G) Herpes simplex.** Herpes genitalis in most cases is caused by herpes simplex virus (HSV) type 2. It can be primary, recurrent, or non-primary first episode. Those with the primary infection present with painful blisters on the vulva, dysuria, low-grade pyrexia and as in this patient rarely urinary retention.
102. **(D) Crystalline penicillin in labor.** GBS carrier rates vary from 15 to 25% and is associated with preterm labor and neonatal infections. Asymptomatic carriers in the genital tract should be given intra-partum antibiotics while those with the bacteria in their urine should be treated at the time of diagnosis.
103. **(H) Rifampicin and isoniazid.** The treatment of tuberculosis in pregnancy should include rifampicin combined with isoniazid,

ethambutol, and pyrazinamide. Streptomycin is contraindicated in pregnancy as it is associated with 8th cranial nerve palsy.

104. **(K) Varicella zoster immunoglobulin.** When a woman develops chickenpox within 7 days of delivery, she should be given aciclovir if the diagnosis is made within 24 hours of the rash appearing and the baby should be given varicella zoster immunoglobulin. It is not a contraindication to breastfeeding.
105. **(A) Aciclovir 400 mg tds.** At this gestation, she should be given aciclovir therapeutically for 5 days. There may be benefit in continuing with suppressive aciclovir until delivery.
106. **(H) Supportive care.** Her symptoms are characteristic of postpartum blues and the management of these include supportive care and if there is significant anxiety and difficulties sleeping, anxiolytics could be prescribed. This patient requires supportive care at this stage.
107. **(F) Psychotherapy and antidepressants.** The symptoms in this patient are in keeping with severe postpartum depression. These symptoms appear usually between 4 and 6 weeks postpartum but may present earlier or later. Precipitating factors include difficult delivery (in this case prolonged labor and forceps followed by an infected perineum). The symptoms are varied and include lack of interest in surroundings the baby, feeling hopeless and feeling worthless, fear of being a good mother, thoughts of self-harm, or harming the baby. Early identification and prompt institution of treatment are vital to prevent progression to adverse effects including suicide/infanticide, physical morbidity, and prolonged psychiatric morbidity.
108. **(A) Admit into mother and baby unit for acute pharmacotherapy.** This woman has puerperal psychosis and this is an emergency that requires urgent referral to psychiatrist or the perinatal mental team. She should be admitted into a mother and baby unit for pharmacotherapy which will include lithium carbonate to start with. Where this fails respond, consideration may be given to electroconvulsive therapy (ECT)
109. **(L) Drug toxicity.** The twitching followed by collapse are features of local anesthetic toxicity. Other features of drug toxicity include headaches and convulsions.
110. **(H) Myocardial infarction.** Myocardial infarction is an important cause of maternal mortality. It can occur at any gestation although it is more common in the third trimester and postpartum. A raised serum troponin is diagnostic. In some cases, creatine kinase is also raised. Characteristic changes on ECG include a new QRS complex and an inverted ST-segment.
111. **(J) Sepsis.** The clinical features are consistent with those of sepsis—pyrexia, warm peripherally, tachycardia, and a wide pulse pressure.

This is more likely from chorioamnionitis since she appears to have ruptured her membranes 3 days previously.

112. **(A) Amniotic fluid embolism.** Amniotic fluid embolism is an emergency that can cause profound and acute respiratory distress in women followed by bleeding diathesis. It results from anaphylactic reaction to the fetal squames in the maternal circulation.
113. **(I) PE.** In this patient, it is likely that she had pelvic vein thrombosis which contributed to the swollen legs. Delivery then removed the pressure of the gravid uterus on the inferior vena cava which would have allowed the clots to be dislodged into the circulation and the lungs. Confirmation of the diagnosis will be with a VQ scan/CT scan.
114. **(E) Lethal fetomaternal hemorrhage.** In this patient, a positive Kleihauer test is indicative of a fetal maternal hemorrhage. This is the most likely cause of the IUFD rather than Rhesus isoimmunization. Although she is Rhesus(D) negative, no antibodies were found antenatally and it is unlikely that even if they developed later, these would be high enough to cause an IUFD. Abdominal pains prior to presentation will suggest a degree of placental abruption.
115. **(I) SLE.** The presence of endomyocardial elastosis is suggestive of heart block which is a complication of SLE. An important investigation in this patient will be anti-Rho and La antibodies.
116. **(C) Gestational diabetes.** Gestational diabetes is an important cause of IUFD. This is more common in those whose diabetes is poorly controlled in pregnancy. In this patient, it seems the diagnosis had not been made but polyhydramnios and macrosomia (both unexplained at this stage will be supportive of the diagnosis of gestational diabetes). A HbA1C will be an important investigation.
117. **(E) Corticosteroids, tocolysis, and magnesium sulfate.** This patient is most likely to progress to deliver. She should therefore be commenced on corticosteroids and tocolysis in the hope that this will delay delivery and give time for the corticosteroids to have a maximum benefit on the fetus. As she is between 24 and 32 weeks the baby will benefit from magnesium sulfate for neuroprotection.
118. **(M) Speculum examination.** The diagnosis needs to be confirmed first before further management. The first step to take will be performing a speculum examination and only if this is inconclusive will other tests such as the Partum™ test be considered.
119. **(B) Cervical cerclage at 14–16 weeks.** Indications for cervical cerclage include history, ultrasound diagnosis of a short cervix or rescue cerclage in women presenting with dilatation and or shortening of the cervix with bulging membranes. In this patient, her past gynecological history of a cone biopsy is considered an indication for a cerclage and the best time to insert this is between 14 and 16 weeks.

120. **(F) Expectant management and deliver after 24–48 hours.** Preterm labor rupture of membranes presenting at 36 weeks or more should be managed expectantly for 24–48 hours and if labor does not start spontaneously it should be induced.
121. **(A) Emergency CS.** Removal of cervical cerclage is indicated if there is vaginal bleeding, rupture of fetal membranes or labor. However, this is only indicated in those where vaginal delivery is possible. Where an interval cervical cerclage has been inserted as in this patient, contractions, bleeding, or rupture of membranes is an indication for CS.
122. **(L) Rescue cerclage.** Indications for cervical cerclage include history, ultrasound diagnosis of a short cervix or for rescue cerclage in women presenting with dilatation and or shortening of the cervix with bulging membranes. In this patient, bulging membranes with a cervix dilated to 2 cm are an indication for a rescue cerclage.
123. **(K) Remove cerclage at 37–38 weeks.** The timing of removal of cervical cerclage is determined by the clinical presentation—where the patient presents with bleeding, rupture of membranes, or contractions this should be removed as an emergency but where the pregnancy progresses without any problems the stitch should be removed at 37–38 weeks.
124. **(C) Compression duplex Doppler of the legs.** The investigation of choice for suspected DVT is compression duplex ultrasound. If this is negative but clinical suspicion remains, this should be repeated after 3 and 7 days.
125. **(A) CXR.** If a woman presents with features of a PE with no signs of DVT, she will require either a V/Q scan or CT pulmonary angiography (CTPA) to confirm the diagnosis. Before this is performed, a CXR should be performed and only when this is normal should she be offered a V/Q scan. If the CXR is abnormal then a CTPA would be the preferred confirmatory investigation.
126. **(C) Compression duplex Doppler of the legs.** Where a patient presents with a suspicion of PE and there are clinical features of DVT, a compression duplex ultrasound should be performed first. If this is positive then there will be no need for further investigations. It is only when this is negative that a CXR followed by V/Q or CTPA will be required to confirm the diagnosis.
127. **(F) Full anticoagulation with unfractionated heparin.** Treatment of a VTE in pregnancy full anticoagulation. When this is peripartum, it would be better to treat with unfractionated heparin as it has a shorter half-life and is easy to reverse with protamine sulfate compared to LMWH. The disadvantage is its frequency of administration and the need to monitor with therapeutic levels. Furthermore, after >5 days

there is the risk of heparin-induced thrombocytopenia requiring monitoring.

128. **(E) Full anticoagulation with LMWH.** Treatment of a PE or DVT is full-anticoagulation. LMWH is the preferred anticoagulant at this gestation. Its advantages include ease of administration, duration action, no need to monitor with Xa levels and minimal or no impact platelets and bone density.

129. **(D) Omit LWMH for 24 hours before CS.** Anyone on coagulants—prophylaxis or therapeutic must omit the LMWH for a defined period prior having a regional for delivery. For those who are fully anticoagulated on LMWH, this is 24 hours while if this is thromboprophylaxis it is 12 hours.

130. **(C) Omit dose of LMWH 12 hours before induction.** For woman on thromboprophylaxis, it is advised that they omit the last dose of LMWH 12 hours before presenting either in labor or for induction of labor or CS.

131. **(H) Prophylactic LMWH antenatally until 6 weeks after delivery.** This woman is high risk for VTE in pregnancy by virtue of having had a DVT in pregnancy and also on an estrogen-containing contraception. It is recommended that those considered high risk like her should be placed on thromboprophylaxis antenatally and until 6 weeks after delivery.

132. **(H) Prophylactic LMWH antenatally until 6 weeks postpartum.** This woman has four risk factors for VTE including her age, parity, smoking, and high BMI. She should therefore be commenced on LMWH antenatally until 6 weeks postpartum. If she had three risk factors the LMWH would be commenced from 28 weeks until 6 weeks postpartum.

133. **(L) Recommence LMWH 4 hours after removing the epidural catheter.** The LMWH should be avoided for 4 hours following regional analgesia/anesthesia. LWMH should therefore be recommenced in this woman 4 hours after removal of the catheter.

134. **(A) Acute appendicitis.** Acute appendicitis, the most common cause of surgical pain in the abdomen in pregnancy affects about 1:800–1,500 pregnancies. Presentation may be unusual in pregnancy as the gravid uterus displaces the structures laterally. In this patient, however, the presentation is typical—central/periumbilical pain (accompanied by systemic symptoms such as fever, nausea, and vomiting) which later settles in the right lower abdomen.

135. **(I) Labor.** In a pregnant patient especially one in the third trimester, intermittent lower abdominal pains that radiate to the back and not associated with systemic symptoms is most likely labor. In this patient, there is no other cause of the pain. The increased in urinary frequency

is most likely related to the head of the fetus descending into the pelvis. A pelvic examination will confirm the diagnosis in this case.

136. **(F) Degenerating fibroid.** Fibroids are the most common benign gynecological tumor presenting in pregnancy with lower abdominal or localized constant pain. The pain is recurrent and may get worse with pregnancy. Degeneration in the fibroids is the pathology responsible for the pain and treatment is mainly analgesia and supportive care.
137. **(B) Acute cholecystitis.** Gallbladder disease is the second most common cause of surgical abdomen in pregnancy (after acute appendicitis). Cholecystitis presents with colicky abdominal pain which is worse postprandial and associated with nausea. Although the gravid uterus displaces most intra-abdominal organs the signs of cholecystitis in pregnancy are similar to those in nonpregnant women. A positive Murphy's sign is diagnostic in this patient.
138. **(M) Pyelonephritis.** Acute pyelonephritis is more common in pregnancy compared to nonpregnancy. It presents with fever, rigors, and abdominal pain (mainly in the lumbar region). Typically, urine is dark in color and urinalysis reveals red blood cells. The presence of bilateral lumbar tenderness in this patient with the clinical features are highly suggestive of the diagnosis.
139. **(C) Acute pancreatitis.** Acute pancreatitis typically presents with central upper abdominal pain which radiates to the back and is worse after meals associated with systemic symptoms of fever, nausea, vomiting, and diarrhea. The temperature is usually around 38°C with tenderness in the epigastrium. Mild jaundice is a positive clinical feature.
140. **(E) Chorioamnionitis.** Chorioamnionitis can occur in women with intact or rupture membranes although it is more common after rupture of membranes. It presents with maternal systemic and localized symptoms including fever, nausea, vomiting, abdominal pains, and reduced to absent fetal movements. If severe the patient may present with features of shock. Treatment is antibiotics and delivery.
141. **(A) Artificial rupture of fetal membranes.** In this patient, the Bishop score has changed and is now very favorable. As she is not contracting regularly the most appropriate next step is to rupture fetal membranes. Following this she may well start contracting effectively but if this does not happen, she would be started on IV syntocinon.
142. **(H) SC terbutaline.** *This patient is experiencing tachysystole.* In this patient who is contracting more than the normal of 3–4 in 10 minutes, the first step to take is administration of SC terbutaline which will slow or stop the uterine contractions. Induction may continue if the tachysystole is corrected or a CS is performed if this is not.

143. **(D) Emergency CS.** The fetal heart rate has changed with a rise in baseline, reduced variability, and late decelerations. As a pathological CTG, a fetal blood sample should be performed or the baby delivered. As she is only 2 cm dilated a fetal blood sample will be difficult hence the next logical step will be an emergency CCS.
144. **(C) Cord prolapse.** Rupture of membranes followed by fetal heart rate abnormalities especially unrecovering bradycardia is suggestive of cord prolapse. A vaginal examination should be performed to exclude this complication.
145. **(B) Commence on IV syntocinon.** Following rupture of membranes if contractions are effective the cervix should dilate at a rate of at least 0.5 cm/h. In this patient, failure to have dilated by at least 2 cm over the 4-hour period despite regular uterine contractions indicate that these contractions are ineffective. Commencing syntocinon should correct any uterine dysfunction.
146. **(G) OP position.** This defines the vertex with the anterior fontanel anteriorly and the posterior fontanel posteriorly with a vertical sagittal suture. This is characteristic of an OP position.
147. **(J) ROT.** The fetus is in a transverse position as defined by the direction of the sagittal suture. The location of the fontanels determines whether this is left or right. In this case, the occiput is at 9 o'clock hence a right OT.
148. **(H) ROA.** The vertex in this case is in the ROA position as the posterior fontanel is at 11 o'clock and the sagittal suture is in an oblique direction.
149. **(F) Extension.** This is the definition of extension a process which follows internal rotation in the course of delivery
150. **(J) Restitution.** This is the definition of restitution a process which occurs soon as the head of the baby is delivered in a normal laboring woman. It follows the process of extension.
151. **(I) Molding.** Molding is defined as overlapping of the fetal skull bones. It varies from 1+ to 3++ depending on how easy it is to separate the bones. Most cases with 3+ are in obstruction.
152. **(H) Latent phase of labor.** The latent phase of labor is the period from the onset of contractions to active labor. Active labor is diagnosed when the cervix is at least 4 cm dilated and there are regular uterine contractions with cervical effacement and in most cases passage of a show.
153. **(A) Active second stage.**
154. **(A) ARM.** The progress of labor in this patient is slow and therefore intervention is necessary. The option at this stage is an ARM followed by a reassessment after 2–4 hours to determine whether she will require syntocinon. In most cases, ARM is followed by regular contractions.

155. **(H) IV syntocinon.** The escalating steps to correct dysfunctional labor include ARM followed by syntocinon. In this patient, although the cervix has not been assessed to determine progress of labor the fact that she is contacting infrequently and the contractions are short-lasting indicates the need for syntocinon. It would be useful to perform a VE prior to commencing syntocinon though.
156. **(G) Fetal blood sampling.** The features of the heart rate are diagnostic of a pathological heart rate pattern and this is an indication for fetal blood sampling as if the pH is abnormal delivery would be indicated.
157. **(E) Emergency CS.** The fetus is most likely acidotic and delivery should be expedited. As she is only 5 cm dilated and the vertex is still above the spines, the best approach to manage this is an emergency CS. In some cases, if the heart rate is very abnormal, there may be no need for a fetal blood sample but proceeding to CS may be more sensible as performing an FBS may be time consuming
158. **(C) Commence pushing.** This woman is now in the active phase of the second stage of labor and should therefore be encouraged to start pushing. This is defined as the time from onset of involuntary expulsive contractions (manifesting as urges to bear down or push). This phase is 1 hour in multiparous women and 2 hours in primigravidae.
159. **(F) Examination under anesthesia.** In the management of postpartum hemorrhage (PPH), the first step is to ensure that the placenta and membranes are complete, ensure the bladder is empty and rub contractions and administer uterotonics such as syntocinon/syntometrine. If the uterus is contracting and the bleeding is continuing especially in a patient like this without an episiotomy or perineal tear, the next step should be an examination under anesthesia to ensure that there are no vaginal or cervical tears that may be the source of the hemorrhage.
160. **(L) Reassess in 4 hours.** The progress of labor in this patient is normal and therefore she should be reassessed in 4 hours. A normal labor progresses at the rate of cervical dilatation of at least 0.5 cm/h and over a 4-hour periods she dilated from 3 to 5 cm.
161. **(E) Trauma.** Hemorrhage following an instrumental delivery is likely to be secondary to trauma especially when the uterus is well contracted. In this patient who did not have an episiotomy, the most likely source of the bleeding is vaginal or cervical trauma. If she were bleeding from the perineum, this would be very obvious. An examination under anesthesia will identify the source of bleeding. The 4Ts of PPH are Tone, Trauma, Thrombin, and Tissue
162. **(I) Uterine rupture.** The classical presentation of uterine rupture is sudden-onset abdominal pains associated with bradycardia or a pathological fetal heart rate. Risk factors in this patient include her parity

and use of syntocinon. The sudden-onset abdominal pain and fetal bradycardia are highly suggestive of uterine rupture. The collapse is secondary to internal hemorrhage. In some cases, the hemorrhage would also be external.

163. **(A) Amniotic fluid embolism.** Clinical features of amniotic fluid embolism include profound and sudden maternal respiratory distress associated with pulmonary hypertension, sudden-onset fetal distress, and bleeding diathesis. In this patient, precipitating factors include polyhydramnios and syntocinon.
164. **(C) Couvelaire uterus.** Where there is a massive abruption like in this patient, there is bleeding into the myometrium which affects contractility. Following delivery, the uterus remains hypotonic with a resultant hemorrhage that is difficult to control with uterotonics.
165. **(H) Uterine inversion.** Uterine inversion is a complication of the third stage where the fundus of the uterus inverts and depending on the degree may come out of the introitus. Clinically, it presents with clinical features of shock that are not in keeping with estimated blood loss. This shock is from vasovagal attack. The finding of a dimple on the fundus is diagnostic.
166. **(A) ARM and review after 2 hours.** When there is dysfunctional labor and there is no evidence of dehydration or acidosis/ketosis, the first action should be ARM followed by a review after 2 hours and if there is no further progress, i.e., the cervix has not dilated by at least 1 cm, syntocinon should be commenced.
167. **(E) Commence syntocinon and review 2 hours.** Following an ARM, it is recommended that the woman is reviewed after 2 hours and syntocinon commenced if she has not dilated by at least 1 cm (i.e., 0.5 cm/h).
168. **(D) Change position.** The first step to take in managing abnormal fetal heart rates includes changing maternal position from the dorsal to lateral position. This is more so with variable decelerations that are thought to be secondary to cord compression.
169. **(K) IV fluids and paracetamol.** This patient has had a prolonged latent phase and is therefore more likely to be dehydrated. The changes in fetal heart rate may be related to possible dehydration. The first approach is to administer IV fluids and paracetamol as well as mobilize the patient.
170. **(F) Fetal blood sample.** A pathological CTG especially one associated with meconium-stained liquor is an indication for fetal blood sampling. This will allow for a decision to either deliver immediately or continue monitoring with a view to repeating the fetal blood sampling.

171. **(L) SC terbutaline.** Uterine contractions which are considered normal should occur at a rate of 3–4 in 10 minutes each lasting between 30 and 45 seconds. In this patient, the contractions are occurring at a rate of 6–7 in 10 minutes each lasting about 45–60 seconds. This is tachysystole which does not allow enough recovery of uterine perfusion hence the abnormal fetal heart rate. Correction is with SC terbutaline which should hopefully reduce the frequency of uterine contractions.
172. **(I) Emergency CS.** Cord prolapse is common after rupture of membranes. Risk factors include multiparity, preterm labor, polyhydramnios, multiple pregnancies, abnormal lie (transverse or oblique) and presentation (breech or shoulder), congenital fetal abnormality, and unengaged presenting part. The management depends on its timing and the stage of labor. For those not in imminent delivery or in whom a vaginal delivery is most likely to be least traumatic, delivery is best by emergency CS. Filling the bladder or elevating the presenting part will buy time.
173. **(A) Allow labor to progress and conduct an assisted vaginal breech delivery.** A frank breech presentation in a multiparous woman who has delivered bigger (than the currently EFW) babies vaginally and where there is no contraindication to a vaginal delivery is an indication for a breech vaginal delivery. Following counseling, labor should be allow to progress and an assisted breech delivery conducted.
174. **(F) Emergency CS.** The CTG is pathological and since an assisted vaginal delivery cannot be conducted at this stage, an emergency CS is indicated.
175. **(F) Emergency CS.** Cord presentation is diagnosed when the cord is the leading presenting part and fetal membranes are intact. The main risk is prolapse, following rupture of membranes. As long as the membranes are intact, the risk is that of cord compression which is often managed by changing maternal position. In this case, the baby has to be delivered by an emergency CS and she should not be allowed to labor.
176. **(A) CS category 1.** The most likely complication in this patient with preeclampsia is placenta abruption (abdominal pains and fetal heart rate abnormalities). Delivery of the baby has to be quick otherwise further compromise will result in a poor outcome.
177. **(C) CS category 3.** She has already been booked for an elective CS but is now admitted in early labor. She should be delivered, however, there is no threat to either the baby or mother. There is therefore no need to rush to deliver her, however, this needs to be scheduled and performed within a suitable timeframe.

178. **(L) Lift out forceps.** One of the indications for an assisted vaginal delivery is maternal exhaustion in the second stage. A lift out forceps would be appropriate here especially as there is evidence of fetal distress, a ventouse can also be used but as there is the need for a quick delivery, a forceps would be preferred.
179. **(I) Third degree perineal tear—IIIC.** A third-degree perineal tear that involves both the internal and external anal sphincter muscles is IIIC.
180. **(A) Cervical tear.** In this patient, the most likely source of the bleeding is a cervical tear. Although the tear could be vaginal, precipitate labor is usually associated with a cervical and or perineal tear rather than a vaginal tear. All the same she requires an examination under anesthesia
181. **(H) Third-degree perineal tear—IIIB.** A third-degree perineal tear that involves >50% of the external anal sphincter muscles but not the internal anal sphincter is IIIB.
182. **(J) Vaginal tear.** The most likely cause of the PPH in this patient is a vaginal tear. Risk factors for a vaginal tear include prolonged second stage, edematous vagina, and manipulations to deliver. The presence of a contracting uterus indicates that the bleeding is either cervical or vaginal and in this case a vaginal tear is more likely.
183. **(P) Rub uterine contractions.** In the algorithm for managing primary minor PPH, uterine contractions should be rubbed in the first instance in women without perineal trauma. The placenta should be reexamined and the bladder emptied. Uterotonics will be the next step to take if the bleeding is persisting and by this time an IV access should be secured.
184. **(I) Examination under anesthesia.** The source of bleeding in this patient is likely to be in the lower genital tract—either the vagina or cervix. As she is contracting and the perineum is intact, the bleeding would be coming from either the vagina or cervix and this can only be identified at examination under anesthesia.
185. **(S) Syntometrine IM or IV.** Following the administration of rectal misoprostol, if bleeding is continuing then Syntometrine (500 µg of ergometrine combined with 5 IU of syntocinon) should be administered as a bolus slowly IM or IV. If this fails to stem the bleeding, consideration should be given to the administration of IM carboprost.
186. **(L) Intrauterine balloon tamponade (Bakri balloon).** Intrauterine tamponade should be considered when uterotonics fail to arrest bleeding secondary to uterine hypotonia. If the uterotonics induce uterine contractions, it is often an indication that the balloon tamponade will be successful.

187. **(J) Hysterectomy.** A hysterectomy should be considered early in the course of managing severe major PPH. Delay in performing hysterectomies has been blamed for many maternal deaths. In this patient, various agents have failed to stop the bleeding including uterine tamponade. A hysterectomy would be highly recommended especially as the anesthetists are concerned about her stability.
188. **(F) Retained membranes.** The most likely cause of PPH in this patient is retained membranes. Ragged membranes suggest that these were not completely removed. She is most likely to benefit from exploration of the uterine cavity and removal of membranes.
189. **(C) Endometritis.** Endometritis is the most common cause of secondary PPH. It typically presents with secondary PPH, constant lower abdominal pains with or without a low-grade fever, and a discharge (offensive lochia). Delivery in the pool is a risk factor for endometritis.
190. **(I) Uterine atony.** The most likely cause of the PPH in this patient is uterine hypotonia. She has several risk factors for this—induction of labor, fetal macrosomia, and polyhydramnios. Palpation of the uterus will confirm atony which should be managed with uterotonics in the first instance.
191. **(H) Trauma to the genital tract.** In the presence of a contracted or contracting uterus and PPH, the most likely source of the bleeding will be the lower genital tract (cervix, vagina, or perineum). If it is not coming from the episiotomy then an examination under anesthesia will be required to identify the bleeding sites for suturing.
192. **(G) Multiple pregnancy.** Uterine overdistension is a risk factor for PPH. In this patient, multiple pregnancy is a risk factor for her PPH. Other factors that could cause uterine overdistension include polyhydramnios and fetal macrosomia.
193. **(F) Maternal obesity.** Obesity is a risk factor for PPH. This is probably multifactorial including poor myometrial contractility in women who are obese, fetal macrosomia, and the tendency for these patients to have prolonged labor.
194. **(L) Syntocinon augmentation.** Syntocinon augmentation as in this patient is a risk factor for PPH. The total duration of labor was <16 hours and therefore this cannot be classified as prolonged hence unlikely to have been an important risk factor.
195. **(K) Prolonged labor with or without augmentation.** The total duration of labor in this primigravida was >16 hours. A combination of prolonged labor and augmentation significantly increased her risk of primary PPH.
196. **(B) Chorioamnionitis (infection).** The indication for delivery in this patient was suspected chorioamnionitis on the basis of a rising

maternal pulse, fetal heart rate and CRP. Chorioamnionitis is associated with poor uterine contractions and therefore a risk factor for PPH in this patient.

197. **(J) Urinary tract infection (pyelonephritis).** Although urinary tract infections are common in pregnancy, pyelonephritis is uncommon. It is however more common than in nonpregnant women. Pyelonephritis (which is more common in those with asymptomatic bacteriuria) presents with a fever, painful micturition, and chills with tenderness in the loins. The urine is characteristically dark (from hemolyzed blood) and urinalysis will reveal leukocytes, nitrites and red blood cells as in this patient. Prompt institution of antibiotics is followed by quick recovery.

198. **(E) Lobar pneumonia.** The clinical features in this patient are diagnostic of a chest infection and specifically a lobar pneumonia. The main distinguishing feature between bronchopneumonia and lobar pneumonia is the fact that in the latter there is consolidation resulting in dullness on percussion and bronchial breath sounds while in the former there is usually wide distribution of crackles. Rusty colored sputum is secondary from *Streptococcus pneumoniae* infection.

199. **(H) Pulmonary embolism.** Thromboembolism is one of the most common direct causes of maternal mortality. It is most common in the first 2 weeks postpartum. Clinical features include chest pain and dyspnea of sudden onset associated with a fever and low oxygen saturations in air. In some patients, there may be features of a DVT but these may be absent in those with pelvic vein thrombosis as the source of the embolus. The diagnosis will be confirmed by a ventilation/perfusion (V/Q) scan or computed tomography pulmonary angiography (CTPA).

200. **(C) DVT—pelvic.** Venous thromboembolism will present with pain in the pelvis or calf or in the lower back, buttocks, and a temperature as in this patient. Swelling of the legs with associated tenderness and a positive Homan's sign are other diagnostic features, however, their absence does not exclude the diagnosis. A high index of suspicion is essential to prevent mortality from DVTs. A duplex Doppler ultrasound will help confirm the diagnosis although a negative result does not exclude a DVT.

201. **(J) Retracted nipples.** Retracted nipples are common, affecting about 9–10% of women. They cause feeding difficulties like in this patient and treatment is either by using suction devices or applying the Hoffman technique. Breast pumps may be useful if these approaches are unsuccessful.

202. **(H) Mastitis.** Mastitis is an inflammation of the breast—the most common organism being *Staphylococcus aureus*. Clinical features include flu-like symptoms, fever, pain, and engorgement of the breast. Some of the women may be tachycardic as well as pyrexial. Treatment is antibiotics such as flucloxacillin.
203. **(A) Direct maternal mortality.** Direct maternal mortality is defined as death of the woman during pregnancy or up to 42 days after delivery from obstetric complications of the pregnancy, interventions, omissions, and incorrect treatment of chain of events resulting from any of these.
204. **(D) Indirect maternal mortality.** Indirect maternal mortality is defined as death of the mother from a condition which is made worse in pregnancy (i.e., deaths resulting from previous existing disease, or disease that developed during pregnancy that was not due to direct obstetrics causes but was aggravated by the physiological effects of pregnancy).
205. **(B) Early neonatal death.** A neonatal death is defined as the death of a newborn with signs of life (heart rate and breathing efforts) irrespective of the gestational age at delivery. This death is classified as early if it occurs within 7 days of life and late if it occurs from 8 to 28 days.
206. **(C) Fortuitous maternal death.** Fortuitous maternal death is defined as death in pregnancy or after delivery that is from a cause unrelated to pregnancy. Although some of these pathologies may progress faster in pregnancy, these are not considered direct or indirect causes of mortality.
207. **(L) Referral for psychological/psychiatric assessment.** Women who have had FGM, especially when done postinfancy (like this patient) suffer from psychological problems which include anxiety, flashbacks, PSTD, increased incidence of domestic violence, and fear of childbirth. Appropriate counseling in the clinic should be followed by referral to psychologist/psychiatrist for assessment and supportive care.
208. **(B) Deinfibulation around 20 weeks.** Following a review of women who have had FGM at booking, those with a narrow introitus that is not sufficient to permit urination, vaginal examination, and safe vaginal delivery should be referred for deinfibulation around 20 weeks. This can be done under local anesthesia. If this is not done, at this time, then it could be done in the first stage of labor, at the time of delivery or postoperatively if the patient has a CS.
209. **(A) Active management of third stage with or without syntocinon infusion.** Complications to look for in this woman include perineal trauma and PPH. It is therefore crucial that precautions are taken for this including active management of the third stage of labor. Since she has an epidural it is assumed that she will have IV access.

210. **(A) Autosomal dominant inheritance.** In autosomal inheritance, there is vertical transmission (affected parents have affected offspring) while unaffected parents produce normal children (unless there is a spontaneous mutation). An affected parent with an unaffected partner will have 1:1 affected:unaffected offspring. Where both parents are affected the ratio changes to 3:1 affected:unaffected.

211. **(B) Autosomal recessive inheritance.** In autosomal recessive disorders, horizontal form of inheritance is present (normal parents often have more than one affected child). Carrier parents with an affected partner will have 50% of offspring affected and 50% carriers; all children of affected parents will be affected, while carriers with unaffected partners will have 50% of their children being carriers.

212. **(L) Sex-linked autosomal recessive inheritance.** In sex-linked inheritance, more males than females express the recessive phenotype. The disease is usually transmitted by asymptomatic females. A carrier mother has the chance of producing 50% affected sons and 50% chance of carrier daughters. An affected father produces no affected offspring but all her daughters will be carriers and no sons of affected father will inherit the gene (i.e., no male-to-male transmission).

213. **(H) Mosaicism.** A mosaic is an individual with multiple cell lines (genotypes), for example, 45XO/46XX as in this patient. This finding is present in 1% of CVS. If it is confirmed on amniocentesis, then the proportion of cells with each of the genotype will determine the phenotype of the child.

Part D: Single Best Answer Questions

OBSTETRIC HISTORY AND EXAMINATION

1. What does gravidity refer to?

A. Total number of pregnancies (current and previous) that progressed to term

B. Total number of previous pregnancies that progressed beyond 24 weeks

C. Total number of pregnancies (past and current) irrespective of when they ended

D. Total number of past and current pregnancies that progressed beyond 20 weeks

E. Total number of pregnancies that progressed beyond 28 weeks

2. A 30-year-old is booking for antenatal care at 12 weeks of gestation. She gives a history of several pregnancies—the first was 6 years ago and ended with delivery of a baby at 24 weeks that lived for 2 days; the second was a miscarriage at 20 weeks a year later; another was a preterm delivery at 30 weeks (baby is alive) and her last pregnancy was an ectopic pregnancy managed medically. Which of this is correct about this woman?

A. She is G4P1

B. She is G4P2

C. She is G4P3

D. She is G5P1

E. She is G5P2

3. A 28-year-old is booking for antenatal care in her first pregnancy. She gives her last menstrual period as 26th August 202X. Assuming that her periods are regular occurring every 30 days. Using Naegele's rule, what will be her expected date of confinement (EDC) [expected date of delivery (EDD)]?

A. 31/05/202X

B. 31/05/202X+1

C. 02/06/202X

D. 02/06/202X+1

E. 04/06/202X+1

4. Which of these factors in a woman's obstetric history will increase the risk of her having gestational diabetes?

A. Previous fetal growth restriction

B. Previous miscarriages

C. Previous preterm birth

D. Previous unexplained polyhydramnios

E. Previous unexplained stillbirth

5. In the examination of a pregnant woman, which is the best place to check for anemia?

A. Buccal mucosa
B. Conjunctiva
C. Nail bed
D. Palms
E. Under surface of the tongue

6. When is the presenting part said to be engaged?

A. When at least 2/5th have gone through the pelvic brim
B. When at least 3/5th have gone through the pelvic brim
C. When at least 4/5th have gone through the pelvic brim
D. When it is fixed and difficult to move
E. When most of it has done through the pelvic brim

ANTENATAL CARE

7. A 26-year-old books for antenatal care at 10 weeks of gestation. Her BMI is 27 kg/m^2. What would be the recommended weight gain for this woman in pregnancy?

A. 5-8 kg
B. 8–12 kg
C. 7–11 kg
D. 11–16 kg
E. 10–20 kg

8. In the history of women booking for antenatal care, one factor increases the risk of fetal growth restriction and VTE. Which is this factor?

A. Interval between pregnancy >10 years
B. Maternal alcohol intake
C. Maternal age >35 years
D. Maternal age <17 years
E. Smoking

9. During the antenatal care of a primigravida, what routine investigations should be ordered at 28 weeks of gestation?

A. ABO blood group and FBC
B. Antibodies and FBC
C. Hepatitis B serology, FBC, and ABO
D. ABO hepatis and HIV serology and FBC
E. ABO and antibodies, FBC, serology for hepatitis, HIV, and syphilis

10. When is the best time to perform first trimester combined biochemistry and NT scan for aneuploidy?

A. 9^{+0}–12^{+6} weeks
B. 10^{+0}–12^{+6} weeks
C. 10^{+0}–13^{+6} weeks
D. 10^{+0}–14^{+6} weeks
E. 11^{+0}–13^{+6} weeks

11. A woman books for antenatal care at 10 weeks. Which of these factors will not be associated with an increased risk of pre-eclampsia?

A. Age >35 years
B. BMI of >30 kg/m^2
C. Connective tissue disease such as SLE
D. Family history of preeclampsia
E. Interval between pregnancies of 6 years

12. Risk factors for gestational diabetes that should be asked after at booking include all of the following except which one?

A. Age >35 years
B. Family history of diabetes in grandparents
C. Obesity BMI
D. Previous big baby
E. Previous unexplained stillbirth

NORMAL PHYSIOLOGY OF PREGNANCY

13. What important cardiovascular change occurs in pregnancy that affects the definition of anemia in pregnancy?

A. Fall in peripheral resistance
B. Increase in blood volume
C. Increase in cardiac output
D. Increase in heart rate
E. Increase in red cell mass

14. Which clotting factor falls in pregnancy?

A. VII
B. VIII
C. IX
D. X
E. XI

15. With regards to the measurement of BP in pregnancy, which Korotkoff sounds are used for the diastolic BP?

A. Korotkoff I
B. Korotkoff II
C. Korotkoff III
D. Korotkoff IV
E. Korotkoff V

FETAL GROWTH AND MONITORING

16. What is the best way to assess amniotic fluid volume around the fetus during the antenatal period?

A. Abdominal palpation
B. Dye quantification of fluid volume
C. Magnetic resonance imaging
D. Perception by the mother
E. Ultrasound scan

17. At what gestational age is the amount of liquor around the fetus at its maximum?

A. 20–24 weeks
B. 24–28 weeks
C. 28–36 weeks
D. 32–38 weeks
E. 34–38 weeks

18. Which is the best parameter to date pregnancies?

A. Abdominal circumference
B. CRL
C. Femur length
D. Last menstrual period of a regular 28-day cycle
E. Head circumference

19. What is the normal term baseline fetal heart rate as determined by a cardiotocograph?

A. 100–120 bpm
B. 110–140 bpm
C. 120–140 bpm
D. 120–150 bpm
E. 120–160 bpm

20. Umbilical artery Doppler is used to assess impedance against the placenta. The resistance rises as placental function decreases. Which Doppler parameter is associated with the worse outcome for the fetus?

A. Absent end diastolic flow
B. Reduced end-diastolic flow
C. Resistance index above the 95th centile
D. Resistance index below the 5th centile
E. Reverse end-diastolic flow

21. A primigravida attends for her routine antenatal care at 36 weeks of gestation and on clinical palpation the fundal height measures 33 cm. An ultrasound scan is performed and shows that the baby is small with normal liquor volume. A biophysical profile is performed. At what score will the woman be reassured.

A. >3
B. >4
C. >6
D. >7
E. >8

22. What is the definition of perinatal mortality?

A. Number of neonatal deaths (7 days) per the total number of live births
B. Number of stillbirths ≥24 weeks and early neonatal deaths (7 days of life) per the total number of births (live and stillbirths)
C. Number of neonatal deaths (28 days) per the total number of live births

D. Number of stillbirths >24 weeks and neonatal deaths (28 days) per the total number of births (live and stillbirths)
E. Number of neonatal and stillbirths per the total number of live births after 24 weeks of gestation

23. What is the most common cause of stillbirth in high-income countries such as the UK?
A. Congenital malformations
B. Fetal growth restriction
C. Hemorrhage (antepartum or intrapartum)
D. Specific placental pathology
E. Unexplained (idiopathic)

24. What is the commonest cause of maternal mortality in high-income countries such as the UK?
A. Cardiac disease
B. Hemorrhage
C. Hypertensive disorders
D. Sepsis
E. VTE

25. What is the most common cause of maternal mortality in low-income countries?
A. Cardiac disorders
B. Hemorrhage
C. Hypertensive disorders (preeclampsia and eclampsia)
D. Intrapartum complications (e.g., ruptured uterus and obstructed labor)
E. Sepsis

PRENATAL DIAGNOSIS AND MANAGEMENT

26. In which of these pregnancy outcomes are the highest number of structural abnormalities likely to be found?
A. Children with learning disabilities
B. Fetal growth restriction
C. IUFDs
D. Preterm births
E. Spontaneous miscarriages

27. Screening for aneuploidy (chromosomal abnormalities is performed in the first trimester by a combination of ultrasound scan and biochemistry. Which of these is not included in the ultrasound screening for aneuploidy?
A. Ductus venosus Doppler
B. Nasal bone
C. Nuchal fold
D. NT
E. Tricuspid regurgitation

28. **Which biochemical marker for aneuploidy is increased in the first trimester in babies likely to have Down syndrome?**
   A. Alpha-fetoprotein (AFP)
   B. Pregnancy-associated plasma protein A (PAPP-A)
   C. Inhibin B
   D. Unconjugated estriol
   E. Human chorionic gonadotropin (hCG)

29. **Which of the following is not considered a normal variant when reporting ultrasound scan findings from an anomaly scan?**
   A. Choroid plexus cyst
   B. Dilated cisterna magna
   C. Echogenic bowel
   D. Echogenic foci in the heart
   E. Two vessel cord

30. **With regards to ultrasound diagnosis of structural abnormalities, which is the abnormality with the highest antenatal detection rate?**
   A. Anencephaly
   B. Cleft lip and palate
   C. Exomphalos
   D. Gastroschisis
   E. Open spina bifida

31. **Which test in the late first trimester will give a high detection rate for Down syndrome with minimal risk to the fetus?**
   A. Amniocentesis
   B. Biochemistry combined with NT measurement
   C. CVS
   D. NIPD
   E. NIPT

32. **What is the recommended cutoff for high risk of Down syndrome from a combined biochemical and NT measurement at 11^{+0}–13^{+6} weeks of gestation?**
   A. 1:100
   B. 1:150
   C. 1:200
   D. 1:250
   E. 1:300

33. **Which of this is not included in the quadruple test that is performed for aneuploidy screening at 14^{+2}–20^{+0} weeks of gestation?**
   A. AFP
   B. hCG
   C. Inhibin A
   D. PAPP-A
   E. Unconjugated estriol

34. **A mother of three has been to the clinic to book for her fourth pregnancy. She had a baby with trisomy 18 in her last pregnancy and lost the pregnancy at 24 weeks. She is very anxious and wishes to know whether this baby is affected or not as she would terminate the pregnancy if the baby is affected. She is now 10 weeks. What would be the best test to offer this woman?**

A. Amniocentesis at 15 weeks
B. CVS at 11–13 weeks
C. Combined NT measurement and biochemistry at 11–13 weeks
D. NIPD at 11–13 weeks
E. NIPT now

35. What is the main disadvantage of CVS over amniocentesis?

A. Higher failure rate
B. Higher infection rate
C. Increased risk of mosaicism
D. Later results from culture
E. Timing of the procedure

MULTIPLE PREGNANCY

36. What proportion of twin pregnancies is dizygotic (from two eggs and two sperms)?

A. 40%
B. 50%
C. 60%
D. 70%
E. 80%

37. What is the most reliable marker for diagnosing MC twin pregnancies by ultrasound scan?

A. Present of a thick membrane between sacs
B. Presence of two gestational sacs
C. Absence of a twin-peak sign
D. Identical gender
E. One placenta

38. An early ultrasound is performed at about 12 weeks in a primigravida (whose periods are irregular) who is found to have a twin pregnancy. The CRL of the twins are significantly different by about 2 weeks. How should the pregnancies be dated?

A. From the mean measurement of abdominal circumference of both twins
B. From the mean measurement of head circumference of both twins
C. From the measurement of CRL of the larger twin
D. From the measurement of CRL of the smaller twin
E. From the mean measurement of the CRLs of both twins

39. What is the most common complication of twin pregnancies?

A. Fetal growth restriction
B. Intrauterine death of one twin
C. Preterm delivery
D. Pregnancy-induced hypertension
E. Vanishing twin

40. Which complication in MC twin pregnancies is associated with polyhydramnios/oligohydramnios sequence where the bladder of one fetus may not be clearly seen?

A. Selective fetal growth restriction
B. Twin-to-twin transfusion syndrome (TTTS)
C. TAPS
D. Twin reversal arterial perfusion sequence
E. Discordant growth

41. When is it best to deliver an uncomplicated MC/DA twin pregnancy?

A. 33–35 weeks
B. 34–36 weeks
C. 35–37 weeks
D. 36–38 weeks
E. 37–39 weeks

42. What is the most common presentation of twin pregnancies at the time of delivery?

A. Beech/breech
B. Breech/cephalic
C. Cephalic/breech
D. Cephalic/cephalic
E. Cephalic/transverse

43. A multiparous woman with twins has delivered the first twin. When will the delivery of the second twin be considered delayed?

A. If it has not been delivered by 10 minutes
B. If it has not been delivered by 20 minutes
C. If it has not been delivered by 30 minutes
D. If it has not been delivered by 40 minutes
E. If it has not been delivered by 50 minutes

44. A woman is seen in the clinic at 12 weeks and following an ultrasound scan is found to have MC/DA twins. When should monitoring for TTTS start in this woman?

A. 14 weeks
B. 16 weeks
C. 18 weeks
D. 20 weeks
E. 22 weeks

BLEEDING IN PREGNANCY–ANTEPARTUM HEMORRHAGE

45. When will bleeding in pregnancy be labeled antepartum hemorrhage?

A. If it occurs after 18–20 weeks of gestation
B. If it occurs after 20–24 weeks of gestation
C. If it occurs after 24–28 weeks of gestation
D. If it occurs from 28 weeks of gestation
E. If it occurs after the first trimester

46. A woman attends for her detailed ultrasound scan at 20 weeks and the placenta is said to be low lying and about 1.5 cm from the internal os. In what proportion of women will the placenta remain low at follow-up ultrasound scan at 32 weeks of gestation?

A. <3%
B. 5%
C. 10%
D. 15%
E. 20%

47. Which of the following is not a risk factor for placenta previa?

A. High parity
B. Maternal age >35 years
C. Multiple pregnancy
D. Polyhydramnios
E. Smoking

48. A 30-year-old multiparous woman presents at 34 weeks of gestation with painless vaginal bleeding for the past 6 hours. The bleeding was initially heavy but is now settling. When examined the abdomen is soft and the fundal height is compatible with gestation. A CTG is reactive. What is the most likely diagnosis?

A. Cervical erosion
B. Cervicitis
C. Placental abruption
D. Placental previa
E. Vaginitis

49. A 28-year-old presents with mild painless vaginal bleeding at 32 weeks of gestation. What would be the next most useful step to take after a general physical examination if the patient is clinically stable (normal pulse and BP)?

A. Blood for group and safe
B. Digital examination
C. Maternal blood for Kleihauer test
D. Speculum examination
E. Ultrasound sound to localize the placenta

50. A multiparous woman has been diagnosed with moderate placental abruption at 37 weeks and on this basis is being induced. What is the most common complication that she may have postdelivery?

A. Acute renal failure
B. DIC
C. Hypertension
D. PPH
E. Retained placenta

51. When should a woman with vasa previa diagnosed at 20 weeks and confirmed at 28 weeks ultrasound scan be delivered?

A. 30–32 weeks
B. 32–34 weeks
C. 34–36 weeks
D. 36–38 weeks
E. 38–40 weeks

HYPERTENSIVE DISORDERS OF PREGNANCY

52. How common are hypertensive disorders of pregnancy (i.e., what proportion of pregnant women suffer with hypertensive disorders of pregnancy)?

A. 1:5
B. 1:6
C. 1:10
D. 1:15
E. 1:20

53. Preeclampsia is defined as pregnancy induced hypertension and either significant proteinuria or hematological/biochemical changes associated with the condition. What is significant proteinuria?

A. Proteinuria of at least 100 mg/24 hours
B. Proteinuria of at least 200 mg/24 hours
C. Proteinuria of at least 3+ in spot urinalysis
D. Urine protein creatinine ratio of >25 μg/mL
E. Urine protein creatinine ratio of >35 μg/mol

54. Among the risk factors for preeclampsia is interpregnancy interval. What interpregnancy interval is considered a risk factor?

A. Interpregnancy interval of <6 months
B. Interpregnancy interval of at least 36 months
C. Interpregnancy interval of at least 48 months
D. Interpregnancy interval of at least 60 months
E. Interpregnancy interval of at least 120 months

55. Which physiological maladaptation is associated with the development of preeclampsia?

A. Abnormal trophoblastic invasion of spiral arteries
B. Decrease production of nitrous oxide
C. Decreased production of thromboxane
D. Increase production of vascular endothelial growth factor (VEGF)
E. Reduced production of placental growth factor (sft1)

56. What does the acronym HELLP stand for?

A. Hypertension and low platelets
B. Hypertension, elevated liver enzymes, and low platelets
C. Hypertension, elevated liver enzymes and proteinuria
D. Hypertension elevated liver enzymes, proteinuria and low platelets
E. Hypertension, proteinuria and low platelets

57. A 32-year-old primigravida is seen at 30 weeks of gestation. Her BP is 150/105 mm Hg on two occasions. She is asymptomatic and her urinalysis is negative for protein. A decision is taken to start her on antihypertensives. Which is the first option for her BP control?

A. Alpha-methyldopa
B. Atenolol
C. Hydrazaline
D. Labetalol
E. Nifedipine

58. What should be offered to a 24-year-old primigravida who is considered high risk for developing preeclampsia based on her medical condition (SLE) and family history of preeclampsia? She is now 10 weeks.

A. Aspirin from 12 weeks
B. Aspirin, vitamin C and E
C. Calcium supplementation
D. Low molecular weight heparin
E. Vitamin C and E

DIABETES AND ENDOCRINE DISORDERS OF PREGNANCY

59. A 31-year-old with type 1 diabetes on insulin attends the pre-pregnancy counseling clinic at her General Practitioner's surgery. She requests for a HbA1C test. At what level would you not advice pregnancy?

A. ≥6.0%
B. ≥7.0%
C. ≥8.0%
D. ≥9.0%
E. ≥10.0%

60. What is the most likely complication in a 28-year-old with Type II diabetes who is now 30 weeks pregnant and has been struggling with her diabetic control and is breathless?

A. Antepartum hemorrhage
B. Congenital malformations
C. Fetal growth restriction
D. Polyhydramnios
E. Spontaneous preterm labor

61. A 28-year-old booked for antenatal care at 13 weeks of gestation. In view of her high BMI, she had an OGTT at 26 weeks of gestation. The results are as follows: Fasting 100 mg/dL (5.6 mmol/L), 1 hour 195 mg/dL (10.8 mmol/L), and 2 hours 154 mg/dL (8.6 mmol/L). A diagnosis of gestational diabetes is made. What would be the first approach in her management?

A. Dietary modification
B. Diet modification and metformin
C. Diet modification and insulin
D. Insulin
E. Metformin

62. How often should a woman with type I diabetes monitor her blood glucose levels during pregnancy?

A. Fasting
B. Fasting and 1 or 2 hours postmeals
C. Fasting and postmeals

D. Premeals, fasting, and postmeals
E. Premeals, fasting, and 1 or 2 hour post meals

63. When would you recommend that a 26-year-old primigravida with Type II diabetes that is well controlled is delivered?

A. $36–37^{+6}$ weeks
B. $37–38^{+6}$ weeks
C. $38–39^{+6}$ weeks
D. $39–40^{+6}$ weeks
E. $40–41^{+6}$ weeks

64. When should women with gestational diabetes that is well controlled diabetes be delivered?

A. Around 36–37 weeks
B. Around 37–38 weeks
C. Around 38–39 weeks
D. Around 39–40 weeks
E. 40–41 weeks

OTHER ENDOCRINE DISORDERS OF PREGNANCY

65. Which of the following is not a complication of thyrotoxicosis in pregnancy?

A. Congenital malformations
B. Fetal growth restriction
C. Miscarriage
D. Neonatal thyrotoxicosis
E. Preterm labor

66. What is the most common clinical feature of hypothyroidism in pregnancy?

A. Asymptomatic
B. Constipation
C. Fatigue
D. Poor tolerance to cold
E. Weight gain

DERMATOLOGICAL DISORDERS OF PREGNANCY

67. A primigravida who is 30 weeks pregnant comes to the emergency complaining of itching and a rash over her body of 3 days duration. Her mother and sister had similar problems in pregnancy and her brother suffers from asthma. When examined she is found to have an erythematous rash on her face, neck, chest, trunk, and the extensor surfaces of the limbs. There are areas of excoriation most likely from scratching on these rashes. What is the most likely diagnosis?

A. Atopic eruption of pregnancy
B. Dermatographism
C. Obstetric cholestasis
D. Pemphigoid gestationis
E. PEP

68. A primigravida who is carrying twins presents at 35 weeks of gestation with itching of the skin and a rash. The rash started on the abdomen and has now spread to the trunk and the limbs but does not affect the palms and soles. Pregnancy has so far been uncomplicated. Physical examination shows an erythematous papular rash distributed on the anterior abdomen located mainly within striae and sparing the umbilicus as well as over the trunk and the limbs. What is the most likely diagnosis?

A. Atopic eruption of pregnancy
B. Dermatographism
C. Obstetric cholestasis
D. Pemphigoid gestationis
E. Polymorphic eruption of pregnancy (PEP)

69. A 30-year-old presents at 34 weeks of pregnancy with a rash which has developed over the last one week. The rash which started around the umbilicus has now spread to involve the trunk, limbs and the palms and soles. On examination there are urticarial rashes on the anterior abdomen and large tense blisters at the edges of the rash. The rashes are also on the trunk, the limbs, and the palms. What is the most likely diagnosis?

A. Atopic eruption of pregnancy
B. Dermatographism
C. Obstetric cholestasis
D. Pemphigoid gestationis
E. PEP

RESPIRATORY DISORDERS OF PREGNANCY

70. What proportion of women is affected by asthma in pregnancy?

A. <5%
B. 5–10%
C. 10–15%
D. 15–20%
E. 20–25%

71. A woman who has been suffering from asthma since she was a child wishes to become pregnant. She is worried about the effect of the asthma on the pregnancy. If her asthma remains well controlled, what would be the impact of it on the pregnancy?

A. Increased risk of fetal growth restriction
B. Increased risk of hypertension in pregnancy
C. Increased risk of preeclampsia
D. Increased risk of preterm labor
E. No impact on the pregnancy

72. What is the effect of pregnancy on asthma?

A. About two-thirds will get better
B. A half of cases will get better

C. A third will remain unchanged
D. Has no effect
E. Two-thirds of cases will get worse

73. A 30-year-old asthmatic on a long-acting beta-2 agonist is in labor. What medication should be avoided in this woman during her labor?
A. Corticosteroids
B. Ergometrine
C. Labetalol
D. Nifedipine
E. Oxytocinon

74. What is the most likely diagnosis in a woman who presents at 30 weeks of gestation with a productive cough, chest pain, fever, and loss of appetite of 3 days duration? On physical examination her temperature is 38.5°C, pulse 95 bpm, and BP 130/75 mm Hg. The chest is symmetrical with a central trachea and localized bronchial breath sounds on the lower right zone.
A. Bronchopneumonia
B. Lobar pneumonia
C. Pulmonary embolism
D. Upper respiratory tract infection
E. Viral chest infection such as influenza

75. What is the most common mutation responsible for CF in the general population?
A. A455E
B. D1152H
C. G542X
D. G551D
E. ΔF508

CONNECTIVE TISSUE DISORDER OF PREGNANCY

76. A 33-year-old woman with SLE has been investigated prior to pregnancy and has been found to have anti-Ro/La antibodies. What complication is unique to these antibodies?
A. Fetal growth restriction
B. Heart block
C. Preeclampsia
D. Preterm labor
E. Recurrent miscarriages

77. A 31-year-old who has had three miscarriages and is now 8 weeks pregnant had been diagnosed with APS. What should she be given to improve the chances of a successful pregnancy?
A. Aspirin
B. Aspirin, a progestogen, and low molecular weight heparin
C. Aspirin and folic acid
D. Aspirin and low molecular weight heparin
E. Aspirin, prednisolone, and low molecular weight heparin

78. Connective tissue disorders such as SLE, APS, and systemic scleroderma are associated with an increased risk of VTE. How long after a normal vaginal delivery should a 32-year-old woman with a connective tissue disease continue with low molecular weight heparin?

A. 7 days
B. 10 days
C. 14 days (2 weeks)
D. 42 days (6 weeks)
E. 84 days (12 weeks)

CARDIAC DISORDERS IN PREGNANCY

79. Heart diseases in pregnancy are classified based on the New York Heart Association (NYHA) classification. What is NYHA class II?

A. Heart disease and inability to carry out any physical activity without discomfort
B. Heart disease with limitation to physical activity
C. Heart disease with marked limitation to physical activity
D. Heart disease with no limitations to physical activity
E. Heart disease with slight limitation of physical activity

80. A woman with Class II NYHA cardiac disease goes into spontaneous labor at 39 weeks of gestation following an uncomplicated pregnancy. How will the second and third stages of labor be managed?

A. Allow normal delivery of first stage and physiological third stage
B. Allow normal delivery and Syntometrine for third stage
C. Shorten second stage with instrumental delivery and physiological third stage
D. Shorten second stage with instrumental delivery and oxytocin for third stage
E. Shorten second stage with instrumental delivery and Syntometrine for third stage

81. How long should a woman with the NYHA Class III be on thromboprophylaxis with low molecular weight heparin after a vaginal delivery?

A. 7 days
B. 10 days
C. 14 days
D. 42 days (6 weeks)
E. 3 months

82. Which of the following is not an important risk factor for peripartum cardiomyopathy?

A. Ethnicity
B. Extremes of reproductive age
C. High salt intake
D. Infertility treatment
E. Malnutrition

83. **Which is the most common type of cardiomyopathy in pregnancy?**
   A. Arrhythmogenic
   B. Dilated
   C. Left ventricular noncompaction
   D. Restrictive
   E. Takotsubo

84. **Which of these is inherited as an autosomal dominant condition?**
   A. Arrhythmogenic cardiomyopathy
   B. Hypertrophic cardiomyopathy
   C. Marfan syndrome
   D. Restrictive cardiomyopathy
   E. Takotsubo cardiomyopathy

RENAL TRACT DISORDERS IN PREGNANCY

85. **How common is asymptomatic bacteriuria in pregnancy?**
   A. Affects <5% of women
   B. Affects 2–10% of women
   C. Affects 10–15% of women
   D. Affects 15–20% of women
   E. Affects 20–25% of women

86. **Untreated, what proportion of asymptomatic bacteriuria will progress to pyelonephritis in pregnancy?**
   A. 10%
   B. 15%
   C. 20%
   D. 30%
   E. 40%

87. **Which organism is responsible for most urinary tract infections in pregnancy?**
   A. *Escherichia coli*
   B. *Klebsiella* spp.
   C. Group B hemolytic *Streptococcus*
   D. *Pseudomonas* spp.
   E. Proteus mirabilis

88. **What is the recommendation with regards to waiting time before trying for a pregnancy after a renal transplant?**
   A. 6 months
   B. 6–12 months
   C. 12–24 months
   D. 18–36 months
   E. 24 months

89. **A 37-year-old who had a renal transplant 12 months ago wishes to start a family. She has attended for a review. Assuming that she is on minimal immunosuppressants that are not teratogenic and there is no evidence of rejection, what should be reviewed prior to her starting to try for pregnancy?**

A. BP, medications, renal function (creatinine), and proteinuria
B. Infections with CMV and *Streptococcus*, and BP
C. Infections with CMV and *Streptococcus*, proteinuria, and BP
D. Renal function, proteinuria, and BP
E. Vaccination against *Streptococcus*, BP proteinuria, and medication

INFECTIONS IN PREGNANCY

90. Which of these infections in pregnancy is associated with microcephaly?

A. Coronavirus
B. CMV
C. Parvovirus B19
D. Syphilis
E. Varicella Zoster

91. It is known that some infections confer lifelong immunity and the presence of antibodies to these infections is used to identify women who are not susceptible to these in pregnancy. Which of the infections below confers lifelong immunity?

A. CMV
B. Herpes virus
C. Influenza
D. Syphilis
E. Varicella zoster

92. Which is the most common viral infection in pregnancy?

A. CMV
B. Hepatitis B
C. Herpes simplex
D. Influenza
E. Parvovirus B19

93. A mother who is a teacher reports contact with a child in her class with chickenpox. She is now 20 weeks. When is the child likely to have been infectious?

A. 24 hours before the rash and 7 days after
B. 24 hours before the rash and until it has crusted
C. 48 hours before the rash and until it has crusted
D. 48 hours before the rash and 7 days after
E. 7 days from the onset of the rash

94. Which infection is the most common cause of nonimmune fetal hydrops?

A. CMV
B. Herpes simplex
C. Parvovirus B19
D. Toxoplasmosis
E. Varicella Zoster

95. A primigravida attends with painful blisters on her vulva of 4 days duration. These are examined and are thought to be herpetic. What investigation(s) should be performed on this patient?

A. Fluid from blisters for polymerase chain reaction (PCR)
B. Fluid from blisters for PCR and dark field microscopy as well as culture and sensitivity
C. Fluid from blisters for viral PCR and then screen for other sexually transmitted infections (STIs)
D. High vaginal and endocervical swabs for microbiology and virology
E. Swabs from the vagina and cervix for viral PCR

96. A woman who has booked for antenatal care has been screened for hepatitis B virus (HBV). Which result will be associated with the greatest risk of vertical transmission of the virus to the fetus?
A. HBV c antigen positive and antibody negative
B. HBV c antigen positive and antibody positive
C. HBV e antigen negative and c positive
D. HBV e antigen positive, and e antibody negative
E. HBV s antigen positive and s antigen negative

97. For an HIV positive woman, at what viral load should she be allowed to delivery vaginally?
A. <50 ribonucleic acid (RNA) copies/mL
B. <75 RNA copies/mL
C. <100 RNA copies/mL
D. <150 RNA copies/mL
E. <200 RNA copies/mL

98. What disease is caused by severe acute respiratory syndrome coronavirus-2 (SARS-CoV-2)?
A. Coronavirus disease-2019 (COVID-19)
B. Middle East respiratory syndrome
C. Bird flu
D. Swine flu
E. Influenza

99. When is infection with *Toxoplasma gondii* (*T. gondii*) likely to pose the greatest risk to the fetus?
A. In the first trimester
B. In the second trimester
C. In the third trimester
D. Intrapartum and immediately postpartum
E. Just before pregnancy

100. Which of these infections are transmitted from domestic animals?
A. Coronavirus
B. Listeriosis
C. Middle East respiratory virus
D. Toxoplasmosis
E. Zika virus

101. A woman is booking for antenatal care and has been offered screening for syphilis. The initial screening test is positive. What would be the next test to undertake to confirm that she has an infection with *Treponema pallidum* (the spirochaete that causes syphilis)?

A. Dark-field microscopy
B. PCR on a blood sample
C. Rapid plasma reagin (RPR) test
D. Treponema pallidum hemagglutination assay (TPHA)
E. Venereal disease research laboratory (VDRL) test

102. Which drug used to treat pulmonary tuberculosis is contraindicated in pregnancy?

A. Ethambutol
B. Isoniazid
C. Pyrazinamide
D. Rifampicin
E. Streptomycin

103. A mother had a spontaneous vaginal delivery 5 days ago. She was discharged home 2 days later. She reports that the baby has sticky eyes which are examined and found to be inflamed with a purulent discharge. What is the most likely cause of the baby's sticky eyes?

A. *Chlamydia trachomatis*
B. *Escherichia coli*
C. Groups A hemolytic *Streptococcus*
D. Group B hemolytic *Streptococcus*
E. *Neisseria gonorrhoeae*

104. How does parvovirus B19 cause hydrops fetalis?

A. By attacking the erythroid progenitor cells leading to anemic heart failure
B. By infecting the placenta and causing placentomegaly
C. By affecting the central nervous system
D. By affecting multiple systems including the cardiovascular and renal systems
E. By infecting the liver and causing a hepatomegaly

105. A primigravida is seen at 37 weeks with blisters in her vulva. Fluid from the blisters shows that she has herpes simplex infection. If this is primary infection, how will she be managed from now onward?

A. Aciclovir for 5 days and allow pregnancy to progress and delivery as normal
B. Aciclovir for 5 days and deliver by elective CS at 39 weeks
C. Aciclovir for 5 days and offer induction of labor at 39–40 weeks
D. Aciclovir from now until delivery as normal
E. Aciclovir from now until delivery by elective CS at 39 weeks

106. What is the recommended treatment for a woman who has been diagnosed with syphilis at 10 weeks of gestation?

A. IM ampicillin
B. IV ampicillin and azithromycin
C. IM azithromycin
D. IM crystalline penicillin
E. IM crystalline penicillin and consider termination of pregnancy

107. A 30-year-old who presented with flu-like symptoms is investigated and diagnosed with *Listeria monocytogenes* infection. What would be the treatment of choice for this patient who is now 16 weeks.

A. Ampicillin
B. Benzyl penicillin
C. Ceftriaxone
D. Erythromycin
E. Trimethoprim/sulfamethoxazole

108. An investigation was performed on a 30-year-old who presented with painful blisters on her vulva. The results are shown in the Table below. Which of these will be consistent with a nonprimary first episode HSV2 infection?

	HSV1 immunoglobulin M (IgM)	*HSV2 IgM*	*HSV1 immunoglobulin G (IgG)*	*HSV2 IgG*
A	Present	Absent	Absent	Absent
B	Absent	Present	Absent	Absent
C	Present	Absent	Present	Absent
D	Absent	Present	Present	Absent
E	Present	Absent	Absent	Present

PSYCHIATRIC DISORDERS IN PREGNANCY

109. What in a woman's history would be considered the greatest risk of postpartum depression?

A. Difficult obstetric delivery
B. History of depression not related to pregnancy
C. Previous postpartum depression
D. Relationship difficulties
E. Social deprivation

110. What is the estimated prevalence of postpartum depression after childbirth?

A. <5%
B. 5–10%
C. 10–15%
D. 15–20%
E. 20–25%

111. A primigravida complaints of difficulties sleeping, lack of energy and feeling overwhelmed 2 days after a normal vaginal delivery. She does not have any negative feelings toward her baby or self-harm. What is the most likely cause of her symptoms?

A. Mild postpartum depression
B. Postpartum blues
C. Postpartum mania
D. Postpartum schizophrenia
E. Severe postpartum depression

MATERNAL COLLAPSE IN PREGNANCY

112. What is the most common cause of maternal collapse in pregnancy?

A. Hemorrhage
B. Thromboembolism
C. Drug toxicity
D. Sepsis
E. Electrolyte imbalance

113. A 31-year-old is brought to the hospital by ambulance at 32 weeks of gestation having collapsed at home. She is examined and found to have a temperature of 35.3°C, a tachycardia (110 pbm) and a BP of 80/50 mm Hg. She is cold peripherally. A suspicion of gram-negative sepsis is made. What would be the most important initial management step to take?

A. Blood culture and lactate and initiation of broad-spectrum antibiotics covering gram-negative, positive, and anaerobes
B. Rapid administration of fluids and initiation of broad-spectrum antibiotics covering gram-negative, positive, and anaerobes
C. Secure IV access and commence broad spectrum antibiotics covering gram-negative, positive, and anaerobes
D. Blood culture, rapid infusion of IV fluids, and commence on antibiotics covering gram-negative, positive, and anaerobes
E. Rapid administration of fluids and initiation of broad-spectrum antibiotics and plan delivery

114. A patient delivers spontaneously and is now suffering from a severe anaphylaxis for which adrenaline is required. What would be the dose and route of adrenaline to be given to this woman?

A. 1:1,000 IM
B. 1:1,000 IV
C. 1:1,000 SC
D. 1:10,000 IM
E. 1:10,000 SC

INTRAUTERINE FETAL DEATH

115. From what gestational age is an IUFD considered late?

A. 20 weeks
B. 22 weeks
C. 24 weeks
D. 26 weeks
E. 28 weeks

116. A 30-year-old presents at 36 weeks of gestation with absent fetal movements for 12 hours. You suspect an IUFD. What would be the best means of confirming the diagnosis?

A. Absence of pulsation in the umbilical artery on Doppler
B. Absent fetal heartbeat on Sonicaid
C. Absence of fetal heart motion on 2D ultrasound
D. Absent fetal heart rate on a cardiotocograph
E. Failure to pick up the fetal heart with a Pinard stethoscope

117. What is the most important reason for investigating an IUFD?

A. To help parents come to terms with their loss
B. To help plan management of the IUFD
C. To help provide answers and plan care in the next pregnancy
D. To help with counseling and grieving
E. To provide support to the parents

118. When should a Kleihauer test be performed in women presenting with an IUFD?

A. All women irrespective of their blood group
B. Placental abruption is suspected
C. The woman had abdominal pains
D. The woman is rhesus (D) negative
E. The woman presented with vaginal bleeding

PRETERM LABOR AND PREMATURE RUPTURE OF FETAL MEMBRANES

119. A woman is admitted in preterm labor in her second pregnancy. At what gestational age will you classify her as very preterm?

A. 22–24 weeks
B. 24–28 weeks
C. 26–30 weeks
D. 28–32 weeks
E. 30–34 weeks

120. What will a 30-year-old who has had three preterm deliveries be told about her chances of having another preterm delivery?

A. Increased 1.5-fold
B. Increased 2.2-fold
C. Increased 3.7-fold
D. Increased 4.9-fold
E. Increased 10-fold

121. Which of these factors is the strongest predictor of preterm birth?

A. Cervical weakness
B. Low socioeconomic class
C. Previous preterm delivery
D. Smoking
E. Use of recreational drugs

122. A multiparous woman has been referred to the clinic on the basis of her risk of preterm delivery. She has been offered transvaginal ultrasound scan assessment of the cervix at 22 weeks. At what cervical length measurement is her risk of preterm labor significantly high?

A. <25 mm
B. <28 mm
C. <30 mm
D. <35 mm
E. <38 mm

123. A 28-year-old who has had three miscarriages at 14, 18, and 17 weeks of gestation is now 10 weeks. She has been offered cervical cerclage in view of a history suggestive of cervical weakness. At what gestational age should the cerclage be performed?

A. 10–12 weeks
B. 12–14 weeks
C. 14–16 weeks
D. 16–18 weeks
E. 18–22 weeks (depending on cervical length measurement)

124. A 26-year-old primigravida comes to the Obstetrics Emergency at 30 weeks with lower abdominal pains that are intermittent. The pains started about 3 hours ago and are mainly in her lower abdomen and radiating to the back. There has been no leakage of water and the baby is moving well. A general examination is performed and her vital signs are normal. The fundal height is 31 cm and the fetus is lying longitudinally. A speculum examination shows a closed cervical os. What would be the next step in her management assuming that the contractions and persisting?

A. CBC, urinalysis, corticosteroids, and commence on tocolysis with atosiban
B. CBC, urinalysis, corticosteroids, and commence on tocolysis with ritodrine
C. CBC, urinalysis, corticosteroids, and commence on tocolysis with nifedipine
D. Urinalysis, corticosteroids, and start on tocolysis with atosiban
E. Urinalysis, corticosteroids, and start on tocolysis with nifedipine

125. When should magnesium sulfate be given for neuroprotection in a woman presenting with preterm contractions?

A. She is 22–26 weeks
B. She is 24–32 weeks
C. She is 22–32 weeks
D. She is 24–28 weeks
E. She is 24–30 weeks

126. How will rupture of fetal membranes be confirmed in a primigravida who presents at 32 weeks of gestation with a sudden gush of water vaginally?

A. Ferning
B. Nitrazine paper test
C. Oncofetal fibronectin
D. Partus™ test
E. Speculum examination

HEMATOLOGICAL DISORDERS OF PREGNANCY

127. What is the definition of anemia in pregnancy according to the WHO?

A. Hb <100 g/L in the first and second halves of pregnancy
B. Hb <110 g/L in the first half and <105 g/L in the second half of pregnancy
C. Hb <110 g/L in the first and second halves of pregnancy
D. Hb <115 g/L in the first half and <110 g/L in the second half of pregnancy
E. Hb <120 g/L in the first half and <115 g/L in the second half of pregnancy

128. What is the most common type of anemia in pregnancy?

A. Combined folate, iron, and B_{12} deficiency
B. Folate deficiency
C. Iron and folate deficiency
D. Iron deficiency
E. Vitamin B_{12} deficiency

129. A couple has come to the clinic for antenatal care. They are both carriers of the sickle cell trait (the man is HbAC and the woman is HbAS). What would be their chance of having a baby with either HbAS or HbAC?

A. 1:4
B. 1:16
C. 1:32
D. 2:4
E. 3:4

130. Beta-thalassemia is a hemoglobinopathy in which a defective B globulin gene is inherited from parents. It is either major or minor. What is the definition of thalassemia major?

A. Transfusion of at least 4 times per year
B. Transfusion of at least 5 times per year
C. Transfusion of at least 6 times per year
D. Transfusion of at least 7 times per year
E. Transfusion of at least 8 times per year

131. A problem with beta-thalassemia is iron overload. Which system is affected most by the iron?

A. Genital
B. Heart
C. Kidneys
D. Liver
E. Lungs

132. What test should be offered to a couple who are both carriers of sickle cell trait and are worried that their child may be affected. The woman is now 10 weeks.

A. Amniocentesis at 15 weeks
B. Chorionic villus sample
C. Fetal blood sample by cordocentesis
D. None-invasive diagnosis (NIPD)
E. Non-invasive prenatal testing (NIPT)

133. How long after a vaginal delivery should a woman with sickle cell hemoglobin C disease receive low molecular weight heparin thromboprophylaxis?

A. 6–10 days
B. 14 days
C. 21–28 days
D. 28–36 days
E. 36–42 days

134. When should blood group, rhesus type, and atypical antibodies be checked during routine antenatal care?

A. At booking
B. At booking and at 28 weeks
C. At booking and at 36 weeks
D. At booking, 28 and 36 weeks
E. At booking and every 4 weeks

135. How much anti-D should be given to a woman who has had a sensitizing event before 20 weeks of gestation?

A. 50 IU
B. 100 IU
C. 200 IU
D. 250 IU
E. 500 IU

136. A 25-year-old primigravid Rhesus D negative woman has had a normal vaginal delivery of a male fetus at 40 weeks of gestation. What precautions should be taken with regards to her rhesus status?

A. Cord blood for genotype of fetus and administer 500 IU anti-D
B. Cord blood for genotype and if positive check Kleihauer and administer 500 IU anti-D within 72 hours
C. Cord blood for direct Coombs test and administer anti-D within 72 hours
D. Cord blood for Hb genotype, indirect Coombs test, and anti-D 500 IU
E. Check Kleihauer and administer 500 IU within 72 hours

137. Which clotting factors fall in pregnancy?

A. Factor II
B. Factor VIII
C. Factor IX
D. Protein S
E. Protein C

138. What is the impact of pregnancy on the risk of VTE?

A. Increased it 2 fold
B. Increased 2–4 fold
C. Increased 4–6 fold
D. Increased 6–12 fold
E. Increased 15–20 fold

139. When in pregnancy and the puerperium is the risk of VTE greatest?

A. First trimester
B. Second trimester
C. Third trimester
D. From 0 to 2 weeks postpartum
E. From 4 to 6 weeks postpartum

ABDOMINAL PAIN IN PREGNANCY

140. A 30-year-old presents with right-sided lower abdominal pain at 24 weeks of gestation. The pain is constant and not radiating. There is no associated nausea or vomiting. She says that her periods were very heavy before she became pregnant. On examination she is apyrexial and her vital signs are normal. The uterus is 26 weeks size and there is a localized area of tenderness on the right lower abdomen. What is the most likely diagnosis?

A. Acute appendicitis
B. Acute pancreatitis
C. Degenerating fibroid
D. Ovarian cyst hemorrhage
E. Pyelonephritis

141. The patient is a 23-year-old primigravida who is 26 weeks pregnant and complaints of pain which was initially in the center of her abdomen but has now settled on the right side. This is associated with nausea and vomiting. She feels warm but does not shiver. Her bowels open regularly. On examination she is mildly pyrexial (temperature 37.6°C), tachycardic (pulse 100 bpm), and her BP is normal. There is tenderness with some guarding over the right lumbar region. What is the most likely diagnosis?

A. Acute appendicitis
B. Acute pancreatitis
C. Degenerating fibroid
D. Ovarian cyst hemorrhage
E. Pyelonephritis

INDUCTION OF LABOR

142. Which of these is a contraindication to induction of labor at term in a 30-year-old woman?

A. Contracted pelvis
B. Intrauterine fetal growth restriction
C. One previous CS
D. Recurrent antepartum hemorrhage
E. Rhesus isoimmunization

143. Bishop's score is used to assess the cervix prior to the start of an induction of labor. Above what score is the induction-delivery interval less likely to be prolonged (i.e., the cervix will be classified as favorable)?

A. 4
B. 5
C. 6
D. 7
E. 8

144. Which of the following parameters is not used in the Bishop score assessment of cervical favorability for induction of labor?

A. Attitude of the fetal presenting part
B. Cervical dilatation
C. Consistency of the cervix
D. Length of the cervix
E. Station of the presenting part

145. A primigravida attends for her routine antenatal visit at 41 weeks of gestation. Following counseling she elects to have an induction of labor at 41^{+5} weeks gestation. A Bishop's score is 4. When she attends and the score is the same, what would be the best option for induction of labor?

A. Artificial rupture of membranes and IV oxytocinon
B. Laminaria tents followed by artificial rupture of membranes with or without oxytocinon
C. Misoprostol 25 µg given orally followed by artificial rupture of membranes with or without oxytocinon
D. Prostaglandin E2 given as vaginal tablets or gel followed by artificial rupture of membranes with or without oxytocinon
E. IV oxytocinon followed by artificial rupture of fetal membranes once contractions start

146. A multiparous woman is being induced with IV syntocinon. She started contracting regularly 3 hours ago. She now complaints of abdominal pains with sudden fetal bradycardia. What is the most likely cause of these symptoms?

A. Cord prolapse
B. Hypertonic uterine contractions
C. Placental abruption
D. Ruptured uterus
E. Second stage

NORMAL LABOR

147. In a normal gynecoid pelvis, what is the anterior posterior diameter at the pelvic inlet?

A. 10.0 cm
B. 10.5 cm
C. 11.0 cm
D. 12.0 cm
E. 13.5 cm

148. Which of the following is not a recognized type of pelvis?

A. Android
B. Anthropoid
C. Gynecoid
D. Platypelloid
E. Scaphoid

149. Which of these bone pairs does not constitute a suture line on the fetal skull?

A. Frontal and parietal bones to form the coronal suture
B. Frontal and parietal to form the sagittal suture
C. Occipital and parietal bones to form the lambdoidal suture
D. Two frontal bones to form the frontal suture
E. Two parietal bones to form the parietal suture

150. A primigravida is admitted in spontaneous labor at 41 weeks of gestation. She reports rupturing fetal membranes an hour before presentation. When examined, the cervix is 6 cm dilated. The presentation is cephalic with the anterior fontanelle at 2 o'clock position with a plus of moulding and no caput. What is the position of the presentation?

A. Left occipito-anterior
B. Left occipito-transverse
C. Right occipito-anterior
D. Right occipito-posterior
E. Right occipito-transverse

151. A primigravida is in labor at 40 weeks of gestation. She is examined and found to be 8 cm dilated. The presentation is said to be brow (the orbital ridges as well as the anterior fontanelle) are felt. What would be the presenting diameter in this presentation?

A. Occipito-frontal
B. Occipito-mental
C. Submento-bregmatic
D. Suboccipito-bregmatic
E. Suboccipito-frontal

152. With regards to the physiology of parturition, how will you describe normal uterine contractions?

A. Of origin in the uterine fundus and spreading downward
B. Origin from the cornu and spreading laterally and downward
C. Originating centrally and spreading downward and laterally
D. Origin from the lower uterus and spreading upward and downward
E. Origin form the internal cervical or and spreading upward

153. When are labor uterine contractions considered as normal/ adequate?

A. When they occur at a frequency of 2–3 in 10 minutes with each lasting 15–30 seconds
B. When they occur at a frequency of 2–3 in 20 minutes with each lasting 15–30 seconds
C. When they occur at a frequency of 2–3 in 20 minutes with each lasting 30–45 seconds
D. When they occur at a frequency of 3–4 in 10 minutes with each lasting 30–45 seconds
E. When they occur at a frequency of 3–4 in 20 minutes with each lasting 30–45 seconds

154. A multiparous woman is attending for her routine antenatal visit at 38 weeks of gestation. She is examined and the singleton fetus is cephalic presentation. When will this presentation be considered as engaged?

A. At least two-fifths of the head have entered the pelvis
B. The head cannot be palpated per abdomen
C. The head is fixed in the pelvis and cannot be moved
D. The maximum diameter of the presenting part has entered the pelvic brim
E. The vertex reaches the cervical spines

155. A primigravida was admitted in spontaneous labor fours ago at 4 cm dilatation. Fetal membranes were intact. She has been contracting at a rate of two to three contractions every 10 minutes and each of the contractions lasts for about 25–30 seconds. She is examined and the cervix is now 6 cm dilated with intact membranes. The fetal heart rate is normal. What action should be taken now?

A. Artificial rupture of membranes
B. Artificial rupture of membranes and IV syntocinon
C. Artificial rupture of membranes and reassess in 2 hours
D. Reassessment after 2 hours
E. Reassessment at 4 hours

156. A fetal pH has been performed on a multiparous woman in labor because of a pathological fetal heart rate. At what pH should delivery be considered?

A. <7.21
B. <7.23
C. <7.25
D. <7.30
E. <7.34

157. A fetal blood sample has been performed for an abnormal fetal heart rate. At what base excess should acidosis be considered?

A. <−12 mEq/L
B. <−10 mEq/L
C. <−7 mEq/L
D. <−5 mEq/L
E. <−4 mEq/L

158. When is the active second stage of labor said to be prolonged in a primigravida who has an epidural in labor?

A. Pushing for >30 minutes
B. Pushing for >60 minutes
C. Pushing for >90 minutes
D. Pushing for >120 minutes
E. Pushing for >180 minutes

159. A woman who expressed her desire to have a physiological third stage delivered the baby 10 minutes ago. The placenta is still undelivered. After how many minutes should an attempt at managing the third stage physiologically be abandoned?

A. 15 minutes
B. 30 minutes
C. 45 minutes
D. 60 minutes
E. 90 minutes

160. What is the definition of primary PPH?

A. Blood loss of at least 500 mL after delivery
B. Blood loss of at least 500 mL within 24 hours of delivery
C. Blood loss of at least 1,000 mL after delivery
D. Blood loss of at least 1,000 mL within 24 hours of delivery
E. Any significant blood loss after delivery

161. In the assessment of neonates, APGAR scores are used. Which of the following is not a component of the score?

A. Activity
B. Appearance
C. Grimace
D. Oxygen saturation
E. Pulse rate
F. Respiratory effort

162. What is the main disadvantage of administering opioids to women in labor who are close to delivery?

A. Increased risk of aspiration and pneumonitis
B. Increased risk of delayed second stage (poor maternal pushing effort)

C. Increased risk of maternal respiratory depression
D. Increased risk of nausea and vomiting
E. Increased risk of neonatal respiratory depression

163. In which group of patients is it not advisable to administer pethidine as a form of analgesia in labor?

A. Diabetes mellitus
B. Epilepsy
C. Hypertension
D. Obstetrics cholestasis
E. Preeclampsia

ABNORMAL LABOR

164. What is the most common cause of poor progress of labor in a primigravida in labor at term?

A. Abnormal fetal lie
B. Cephalic-pelvic disproportion
C. Dysfunctional uterine contractions
D. Malposition
E. Malpresentation

165. A multiparous woman is in labor at 40 weeks of gestation. Her baby was estimated to weigh 4.8 kg compared to her previous two babies who weighed 2.9 and 3.2 kg. She progressed well initially but has now developed secondary arrest which is thought to be due to cephalopelvic disproportion (obstructive labor). What finding on vaginal examination will support the diagnosis?

A. A high head
B. Caput ++
C. Deflexed occipito-posterior
D. Moulding ++
E. Tight fitting head with cervical edema

166. In a face presentation, what is the presenting diameter?

A. Occipito-bregmatic
B. Occipito-frontal
C. Occipito-mental
D. Suboccipito-bregmatic
E. Suboccipito-frontal

167. What is the definition of precipitate labor?

A. Labor lasting <0.5 hour
B. Labor lasting <1 hour
C. Labor lasting <2 hours
D. Labor lasting <3 hours
E. Labor lasting <4 hours

168. A G2P1, is in labor at 42 weeks of gestation. The fetal head has just been delivered. When will a diagnosis of shoulder dystocia be made?

A. The shoulders have not been delivered after 15 seconds from delivery of the head
B. The shoulders have not been delivered after 30 seconds from delivery of the head
C. The shoulders have not been delivered after 60 seconds from delivery of the head
D. The shoulders have not been delivered after 2 minutes from delivery of the head
E. The shoulders have not been delivered after 5 minutes from delivery of the head

169. When is the placenta said to be retained after a normal vaginal delivery in a primigravida?

A. Failure to deliver it within 15 minutes of delivery of the baby if physiological management of the third stage
B. Failure to deliver it within 30 minutes of delivery of the baby if physiological management of the third stage
C. Failure to deliver it within 45 minutes of delivery of the baby if physiological management of the third stage
D. Failure to deliver it within 60 minutes of delivery of the baby if physiological management of the third stage
E. Failure to deliver it within 90 minutes of delivery of the baby if physiological management of the third stage

170. Which of these is not a risk factor for shoulder dystocia?

A. Diabetes mellitus
B. Fetal macrosomia
C. Maternal age >35 years
D. Maternal obesity
E. Previous shoulder dystocia

ABNORMAL PRESENTATION

171. At which of these gestational ages is breech presentation highest?

A. 28 weeks
B. 32 weeks
C. 34 weeks
D. 36 weeks
E. 40 weeks

172. When should an ECV be performed on a primigravida with a breech presentation at 34 weeks of gestation?

A. 34–35 weeks
B. 35–36 weeks
C. 36–37 weeks
D. 37–38 weeks
E. 38–39 weeks

173. A primigravida attends for her antenatal care at 36 weeks. The pregnancy has been uncomplicated so far. On examination the baby is presenting by the breech. What is the most likely cause of the breech presentation?

A. Congenital uterine malformation
B. Fetal abnormality
C. Idiopathic
D. Pelvic tumor
E. Placenta previa

OPERATIVE VAGINAL DELIVERY

174. Which of the following is a contraindication to an instrumental vaginal delivery?

A. Fetal distress in the second stage
B. Maternal vulva varicose veins
C. Persistent occipito-posterior presentation
D. Preterm <34 weeks
E. Vertex at spines

175. A primigravida is in labor at term. She has been fully dilated for 3 hours and pushing for one of these. She is now exhausted and a decision is taken to assist delivery with a ventouse. A vaginal examination is performed prior to applying the ventouse cup. What important finding will determine the placement of the cup?

A. The adequacy of the pelvis
B. The degree of caput formation
C. The degree of molding
D. The flexion point
E. The station of the presenting part

176. A forceps delivery is being performed for maternal exhaustion. When will the attempt be considered a failed forceps delivery?

A. Failure to deliver of the head after one pull
B. Failure to deliver of the head are two pulls
C. Failure to deliver the head after three pulls
D. The instrument cannot be applied properly
E. The instrument slips off after one pull

177. A forceps delivery has been successfully performed on a multiparous woman who had an epidural on account of fetal distress in the second stage. How long after delivery should a Foley's catheter be left in situ?

A. 1 hour
B. 3 hours
C. 6 hours
D. 12 hours
E. 24 hours

178. A woman has had an emergency CS for fetal distress. She is about to go home and wishes to know about her chances of having a normal vaginal delivery in the next pregnancy. What success rate of vaginal birth after a cesarean section (VBAC) will you give her?

A. 50%
B. 60%
C. 70%
D. 80%
E. 90%

179. Following an emergency CS, what would be the risk of uterine rupture in labor in the next pregnancy?

A. <0.5% (<1:200)
B. 0.5% (1:200)
C. 1.0% (1:100)
D. 1.5% (3:200)
E. 2.0% (2:100)

180. With regard to the timing of elective CSs, why is it advisable not to delivery before 39 weeks of gestation?

A. Increased risk of intracranial hemorrhage
B. Increased risk of intraventricular hemorrhage
C. Increased risk of neonatal hypoglycemia
D. Increased risk of neonatal jaundice
E. Increased risk of transient tachypnea of the newborn (TTN)

EPISIOTOMY AND PERINEAL TEARS

181. Following a normal delivery by a 20-year-old primigravida the perineum is examined and a tear is found. The tear involved the skin, perineal muscles and about 30% of the external anal sphincter muscle. What type of perineal tear does she have?

A. First degree
B. Second degree
C. Third degree category A
D. Third degree category B
E. Third degree category C

182. Following which type of perineal tear should antibiotics be administered for 5–7 days?

A. A mediolateral episiotomy
B. A midline episiotomy
C. All perineal tears
D. All third- and fourth-degree perineal tears
E. Fourth-degree perineal tears only

POSTPARTUM HEMORRHAGE

183. Primary PPH is defined as blood loss of >500 mL of delivery or less if the baseline Hb is low within 24 hours of delivery. This is further classified into minor moderate and severe major hemorrhage. What is considered severe major hemorrhage?

A. Blood loss of >1,000 mL
B. Blood loss of >1,200 mL
C. Blood loss of >1,500 mL
D. Blood loss of >2,000 mL
E. Blood loss of >2,500 mL

184. What percentage of deliveries is complicated by primary PPH?
A. <5%
B. 5–10%
C. 10–15%
D. 15–20%
E. 20–25%

185. What is the most common cause of primary PPH?
A. DIC
B. Perineal tears
C. Retained placenta
D. Uterine atony
E. Vaginal tears

186. A primigravida has just had a normal vaginal delivery followed by controlled cord traction delivery of the placenta. IM syntocinon 5 IU was given with delivery of the anterior shoulder. You have been called to see her as she is bleeding. The estimated blood loss is now 600 mL. What is the next step you will take in her management?
A. Empty the bladder while asking for checking of completeness of the placenta and membranes
B. Repeat syntocinon IM 5 IU
C. Rub uterine contractions
D. Rub uterine contractions while asking for completeness of the placenta and membranes
E. Secure an IV line with two large bore cannulas and send blood for an urgent FBC

187. In the management of primary PPH, when a decision is taken to administer carboprost, how much of this should be given?
A. A total of eight 0.25 micrograms doses
B. A total of eight 0.5 micrograms doses
C. A total of 100 micrograms in eight divided doses
D. A total of 500 micrograms in eight divided doses
E. A total of 2 micrograms in divided eight divided doses

188. What factor is considered to have the greatest risk of uterine rupture in a woman who has had one previous CS and wishes to delivery vaginally?
A. Indication for the previous CS (elective or intrapartum)
B. Prolonged latent phase of labor
C. Prostaglandin induction of labor
D. Syntocinon augmentation of labor
E. Use of intracervical catheter to induce labor

189. A multiparous woman delivers spontaneously and following delivery of the placenta there is a suspicion of an inverted uterus. Which finding is unlikely to be associated with this complication?

A. Dimple in the uterine fundus
B. Hemorrhage
C. Lower abdominal pain
D. Mass in the vagina
E. Well-contracted uterus

190. How long after a normal vaginal delivery does the uterus become a pelvic organ (i.e., is not palpable per abdomen)?

A. 2–4 days
B. 4–7 days
C. 7–10 days
D. 10–14 days
E. 14–21 days

THE PUERPERIUM AND PUERPERAL DISORDERS

191. After how many days does lochia change from red (*Lochia rubra*) which is present after delivery to pink (*Lochia serosa*)?

A. 2–3
B. 3–4
C. 4–7
D. 7–10
E. 10–14

192. In a woman who is not breastfeeding when is ovulation expected to resume?

A. 1 week after delivery
B. 2 weeks after delivery
C. 3 weeks after delivery
D. 4 weeks after delivery
E. 5–6 weeks after delivery

193. Approximately what proportion of women experience perineal pain in the first 3–10 days postpartum following a normal vaginal delivery?

A. 40%
B. 50%
C. 60%
D. 70%
E. 80%

194. When can a woman who has had a CS undertake abdominal stretch exercises?

A. 2 weeks
B. 3 weeks
C. 4 weeks
D. 6 weeks
E. 8 weeks

195. What is the definition of puerperal pyrexia?

A. A temperature of at least 38°C after 24 hours of delivery and up to 14 days
B. A temperature of at least 38.5°C after delivery and up to 14 days

C. A temperature of at least 38°C after delivery associated with tachycardia and up to 14 days
D. A temperature of at least 38°C on more than two occasions after 24 hours of delivery and up to 14 days
E. A temperature of more than 37.5°C postpartum and up to 14 days

196. Which is the organism most responsible for postpartum pyrexia?
A. *Beta-hemolytic streptococcus*
B. *Escherichia coli*
C. *Haemophilus influenzae*
D. *Klebsiella pneumonia*
E. *Staphylococcus aureus*

197. A woman who delivered a few days ago is admitted with genital sepsis. What is the first and most important step to take in her management?
A. Blood for FBC and prompt administration of IV antibiotic covering gram-negative and positive organisms and anaerobes
B. Blood for markers of sepsis (CRP and procalcitonin) and prompt administration of IV antibiotic covering gram-negative and positive organisms and anaerobes
C. Blood cultures and prompt administration of IV antibiotic covering gram-negative and positive organisms and anaerobes
D. Prompt administration of IV broad-spectrum antibiotics covering gram-negative and positive organisms and anaerobes
E. Prompt administration of IV antibiotic covering gram-negative and positive organisms and anaerobes and blood for renal function test

198. Which organism that causes genital sepsis is most likely to require debridement of necrotic tissue?
A. *Clostridium perfringens*
B. *Escherichia coli*
C. *Pseudomonas aeruginosa*
D. *Groups A hemolytic Streptococcus*
E. *Ureaplasma urealyticum*

199. At what serum lactate level will sepsis be considered severe?
A. >2 mmol/L
B. >4 mmol/L
C. >6 mmol/L
D. >8 mmol/L
E. >10 mmol/L

LACTATION

200. Following delivery, when is colostrum replaced by milk?
A. From second to third day postpartum
B. From third to fourth day postpartum

C. From fourth to fifth day postpartum
D. From fifth to sixth day postpartum
E. From sixth to seventh day postpartum

201. What is the main difference between cow's milk and human milk?
A. Cow's milk contains more calories/mL
B. Cow's milk contains more fat
C. Cow's milk contains more lactulose
D. Cow's milk contains more protein
E. Cow's milk contains more water

202. What is the main benefit of colostrum to the newborn?
A. Provides more fat
B. Provides less protein to the baby who is not able to digest these until day 3 of life
C. Provides more immunoglobulins
D. Provides more lactulose
E. Provides more minerals (sodium phosphorus and calcium) needed for the first few days of life

203. There are several benefits of breastfeeding over bottle feeding. Which of this is not a benefit of breastfeeding?
A. Increase risk of juvenile diabetes
B. Reduced risk of atopic dermatitis
C. Reduced risk of childhood asthma
D. Reduce risk of gastroenteritis
E. Reduce risk of necrotizing enterocolitis in preterm and severely growth restricted babies

204. A woman does not wish to breastfeed. What should she be offered as a first measure to help stop lactation?
A. Analgesics and firm bra for 2 weeks
B. Avoid expression, analgesics, and firm bra for 2 weeks
C. Combined oral contraceptive
D. Bromocriptine
E. Cabergoline

205. A woman who delivered her first baby a few days ago has come back with pain in her right breast and fever. She is examined and diagnosed with mastitis. What would be the treatment for this patient who is breastfeeding?
A. Ceftriaxone and acetaminophen
B. Clavulanic acid (Augmentin) and acetaminophen
C. Erythromycin and acetaminophen
D. Flucloxacillin and acetaminophen
E. Penicillin V and acetaminophen

PERINATAL MORTALITY AND MATERNAL MORTALITY

206. What is the definition of perinatal mortality rate?

A. The total number of neonatal deaths per 1,000 total birth
B. The total number of stillbirths and neonatal deaths per 1,000 live births
C. The total number of stillbirths and early neonatal deaths per 1,000 total births
D. The total number of stillbirths and early neonatal deaths per 1,000 total live births
E. The total number of stillbirths and neonatal deaths per 1,000 total births

207. What is the most common cause of stillbirths in high-income countries?

A. Antepartum hemorrhage
B. Congenital malformations
C. Fetal growth restriction
D. Placental pathology
E. Unexplained

208. What is the most common cause of direct maternal death world-wide?

A. Abortions and complications
B. Hemorrhage
C. Hypertension
D. Sepsis
E. Thromboembolism

209. Up to when will the death of a woman who has had a baby be considered a maternal mortality according to the WHO definition?

A. 4 weeks
B. 6 weeks
C. 3 months
D. 6 months
E. 12 months

FEMALE GENITAL MUTILATION

210. A woman comes to book for antenatal care and indicates that she had been circumcised as a child. She is examined and found to have total removal of the clitoris. What type of fetal genital mutilation does she have?

A. Type 1
B. Type 2
C. Type 3
D. Type 4
E. Type 5

211. What will you as consider Type 3 FGM?

A. All procedures that do not involve cutting but include pricking, piercing, incising, scarping, and cauterization
B. Narrowing of the vaginal orifice with the creation of a covering seal by cutting and appositioning the labia minora
C. Partial or complete removal of the clitoris (clitoridectomy)
D. Partial or total removal of the clitoris and labia minora
E. Partial or total removal of the clitoris and labia minora with or without excision of the labia major (excision)

212. A woman who is booking for her antenatal care at 10 weeks of gestation gives a history of genital mutilation as a child. When examined she is found to have a narrow introitus that will not allow a digital vaginal examination. She is counseled and elects to have de-infibulation. When should this be performed?

A. Around 12 weeks
B. Around 14 weeks
C. Around 16 weeks
D. Around 20 weeks
E. Around 28 weeks

213. Which of this is not a complication of FGM in pregnancy?

A. Anxiety
B. Increased risk of stillbirth
C. PPH
D. PTSD
E. Preterm delivery

FASTING IN PREGNANCY

214. What is the risk of fasting in pregnancy by women who do not suffer from diabetes are on a balanced diet?

A. Congenital malformations
B. Fetal growth restriction
C. Miscarriages
D. None
E. Preterm delivery

215. Which of this is not a risk of fasting in pregnancy for women who are diabetic?

A. Difficulties with glycemic control
B. Hypoglycemia
C. Hyperglycemia
D. Ketoacidosis
E. Spontaneous preterm labor

216. A 30-year-old with type II diabetes is now 30 weeks into her second pregnancy. She has been fasting and now presents as an emergency. There is a suspicion that she may be hypoglycemic. What clinical feature is most likely to help distinguish hypoglycemia from hyperglycemia?

A. Abdominal pain
B. Extreme thirst
C. Hunger
D. Nausea and vomiting
E. Sweating and chills

APPLIED GENETICS IN OBSTETRICS

217. A couple attend for counseling about the risk of their child being affected by CF as they are both carriers of the mutation for CF. What should they be told about their children's risk of CF?

A. 50% of the children will be carriers and 50% will be normal
B. 25% of children will be carriers and 75% will be normal
C. 75% of children will be carriers and 25% will be normal
D. All the children will be carriers like their parents
E. 25% will be normal, 29% will be carriers and 50% will be affected
F. 25% will be normal, 25% affected, and 50% will be carriers

218. A mother is a carrier of hemophilia A, a sex-linked disorder. Her partner is normal. What are the risks of this condition to the children?

A. 25% of females are carriers and 50% of males are carriers
B. 25% of males are affected and 25% of females are carriers
C. 25% of males are carriers and 25% of females are carriers
D. 25% of males are affected and 50% of females are carriers
E. 50% of males are affected and 50% of females are carriers

219. During embryogenesis what factor causes the gonads to develop into testes?

A. Anti-Müllerian hormone (AMH)
B. Follicle-stimulation hormone (FSH)
C. Luteinizing hormone (LH)
D. Sex-determining region on Y chromosome
E. Testosterone

220. What is responsible for the development of the Müllerian system in female embryos?

A. Absence of AMH
B. Absence of SRY region on the Y chromosome
C. FSH
D. LH
E. Estrogen produced from the ovaries

Part D: Answer and Explanations

1. **(C) Total number of pregnancies (past and current) irrespective of when they ended.** Gravidity refers to the total number of pregnancies a woman has had including the current pregnancy (i.e., past pregnancies and the current pregnancy). All previous pregnancies are included irrespective of when these ended (i.e., it includes miscarriages and ectopic pregnancies).
2. **(E) She is G5P2.** This woman has had two deliveries—one that was a neonatal death and the other a preterm baby that is alive and well. She then had two other pregnancies one an ectopic and the other a miscarriage at 20 weeks. She is thus in her fifth pregnancy (gravidity 5) and is para 2 as she has had 2 deliveries.
3. **(C) 02/06/202X.** Calculation of EDD/EDC using Naegele's rule consists of adding 7 days to the date and subtracting 3 from the months. Where the total days exceed that for the month, these are moved to the next month. Here 26 + 7 = 33 and for the month 8 – 3 = 5 (i.e., May). But as May has only 31 days the 33 moves into the next month hence the EDD/EDC is 2/6/202x.
4. **(E) Previous unexplained stillbirth.** Risk factors for gestational diabetes include family history, obesity, previous unexplained stillbirth, or fetal macrosomia. A previous small baby is a risk factor for fetal growth restriction.
5. **(E) Under surface of the tongue.** Clinical features of anemia are usually present on inspection of the palms, conjunctiva, buccal mucosa, and the nail bed. Most of the areas are affected by several factors that may make them unreliable. The most reliable place to check for anemia is the undersurface of the tongue.
6. **(B) When at least 3/5th have gone through the pelvic brim.** Engagement is defined as the maximum diameter of the presenting part entering the pelvic brim. This is diagnosed clinically by palpation demonstrating that at least 3/5th of the presenting part have gone through the pelvic brim. A fixed head is not necessarily engaged (analogy of egg in an egg cup) as the head may be fixed when only 2/5th have enter the brim.
7. **(D) 11–16 kg.** For normal weight women the recommended weight gain in pregnancy is 11–16 kg. For overweight women, the recommended weight gain is 7–11 kg whilst for obese women this is 5–9 kg.
8. **(E) Smoking.** Maternal age >35 years is a risk factor for hypertensive disorders of pregnancy (especially if first pregnancy or interval between pregnancy is >10 years), medical disorders such as gestational diabetes,

VTE but not fetal growth restriction. Smoking increases the risk of VTE, fetal growth restriction, and placental abruption. Maternal age <17 years is associated with an increased risk of anemia, molar pregnancy, hypertensive disorders of pregnancy, and small for gestational age.

9. **(B) Antibodies and FBC.** Routine investigations at booking include a FBC, ABO and Rh(D) blood types, antibody screen, serology for HIV, rubella, hepatitis and syphilis, and Hb genotype. At 28 weeks only a FBC and antibodies are measured.
10. **(E) 11^{+0}–13^{+6} weeks.** First trimester combined ultrasound scan and biochemistry screening for aneuploidy should be performed when the crown rump length (CRL) measures 45–84 mm and this is usually at 11^{+0}–13^{+6} weeks.
11. **(E) Interval between pregnancies of 6 years.**
12. **(B) Family history of diabetes in grandparents.** Apart from family history of diabetes in grandparents the other risk factors are associated with an increased risk of GDM. The family history associated with an increased risk is that of diabetes in first-degree relatives (mother, father, or siblings).
13. **(B) Increase in blood volume.** Physiological changes in the cardiovascular system include an increase in cardiac output, fall in peripheral resistance, increase in heart rate, increase in red cell mass, and increase in blood volume. The increase in blood volume is more than the increase in red cell mass and this results in hemodilution. Anemia is therefore defined as Hb <110 g/dL in the first half of pregnancy and <105 g/dL in the second half.
14. **(E) XI.** Coagulation factors VII, VIII, IX, and X increase in pregnancy; II and V remain unchanged and XI falls. Plasma fibrinogen levels increase especially in late pregnancy.
15. **(E) Korotkoff V.** In pregnancy, a fall in peripheral resistance from vasodilation makes it difficult to distinguish Korotkoff IV from V (muffling to disappearance), hence the recommendation is to use Korotkoff V when the sounds disappear.
16. **(E) Ultrasound scan.** Liquor volume can be assessed in several ways; however, the most commonly used tool is quantification by ultrasound scan either by means of amniotic fluid index (AFI) or single deepest pool. Clinical assessment of liquor volume is subjective and unreliable.
17. **(C) 28–36 weeks.** Liquor volume is greatest between 28 and 36 weeks and thereafter the volume falls significantly toward term. The source of amniotic fluid once the fetal kidneys start producing urine is predominantly urine.
18. **(B) CRL.** The most accurate parameter used to determine gestational age is the CRL measured between 7^{+0} and 13^{+6} weeks. It estimates

gestational age with a margin of error of 2–3 days. The head circumference is useful from 14 to 20 weeks and gives an estimate with a margin of error of 6 days. After 20 weeks a combination of head circumference and femur length is used but the accuracy of estimation is higher.

19. **(D) 120–150 bpm.** The normal baseline fetal heart rate at term is 120–150 bpm. However, the baseline can be as low as 110 and as high 160 bpm as long as these are uncomplicated.
20. **(E) Reverse end-diastolic flow.** The resistance index in the umbilical artery falls with pregnancy (meaning the velocity during diastole increases so that the ratio of the systole to diastole falls (i.e., getting closer to 0). An increase in impedance is represented by increase in resistance index. As the diastolic velocity falls, the resistance increases and eventually flow during diastole is absent and then reversed. This is the worst scenario associated with significant perinatal mortality and morbidity.
21. **(D) >7.** A biophysical score of 4 is abnormal requiring action while a score of 6 is equivocal requiring further fetal assessment. A score of 8 (>7) is reassuring.
22. **(B) Number of stillbirths ≥24 weeks and early neonatal deaths (7 days of life) per the total number of births (live and stillbirths).** Perinatal mortality is a marker of maternity care and is defined as the total number of early neonatal deaths (deaths within 7 days of birth) of babies born with signs of life irrespective of gestational age and number of stillbirths (after viability—defined as 24 weeks) per total live and stillbirths.
23. **(E) Unexplained (idiopathic).** Most stillbirths in high-income countries are unexplained. Among the known causes are antepartum or intrapartum hemorrhage, congenital malformations, fetal growth restriction, and specific placental pathologies.
24. **(E) VTE.** In the high-income countries such as the UK the most common cause of maternal mortality is VTE followed by cardiac diseases.
25. **(B) Hemorrhage.** In low-income countries, the most common causes of maternal mortality are hemorrhage and sepsis.
26. **(E) Spontaneous miscarriages.** Congenital malformations affect about 2–4% of all pregnancies. The highest percentage is found in miscarriages (70%) followed by IUFDs (up to 20 weeks) and children with learning disabilities.
27. **(C) Nuchal fold.** Nuchal fold is used in the second trimester. The ultrasound markers are usually the nasal bone, NT, ductus venous Doppler, and tricuspid regurgitation.
28. **(E) Human chorionic gonadotropin (hCG).** First trimester screening includes a combination of biochemistry (hCG, inhibin A, and

PAPP-A but not unconjugated estriol and AFP). Inhibin B is not one of the analytes measured. Inhibin A and hCG levels are high in Down syndrome fetuses while PAPP-A levels are low.

29. **(C) Echogenic bowel.** What are now described as "normal variants" were in the past known as "soft markers" and include choroid plexus cysts, dilated cisterna magna, echogenic focus in the fetal heart, and two vessel cords. Their isolated presence does not require further investigations whereas the presence of echogenic bowel, renal pelvic dilatation, ventriculomegaly, and a nuchal fold (from 16 weeks) of >6 mm require further assessment.
30. **(A) Anencephaly.** The detection rate for anencephaly is highest antenatally followed by that of spina bifida. Detection rates for cardiac abnormalities and skeletal abnormalities are the lowest.
31. **(E) NIPT.** Combined biochemistry and NT measurements generate a detection rate of around 90% whereas NIPT has a detection rate for Down syndrome of 99.9% with a 0% risk to the pregnancy. A CVS will generate an almost 100% certainty of the karyotype, it is associated with a 2% miscarriage risk and 1% of risk of mosaicism. Amniocentesis is in generally not offered until after 14 completed weeks (i.e., from 15 weeks).
32. **(B) 1:150.** The cutoff for invasive testing with the combined NT and biochemical screening test in the first trimester is 1:150.
33. **(D) PAPP-A.** The quadruple test which is performed between 14 and 20 weeks of gestation is a combination of 4 analytes (hCG, inhibin A, and AFP, and uE3). PAPP-A is not measured at this gestation.
34. **(B) CVS at 11–13 weeks.** This woman with a previously affected baby wishes to know definitely whether her baby is affected or not. A screening test is therefore not the best option for her. Although NIPT will provide a diagnostic accuracy of 99.8% for trisomy 18 (Edward syndrome), it is not diagnostic. A CVS is therefore the test to offer her. As she wishes to have a termination, it would be better to have a diagnosis earlier rather than wait until 15 weeks.
35. **(C) Increased risk of mosaicism.** The main disadvantage of CVS over amniocentesis is the higher mosaicism rate with CVS (1%). The timing to results is same and the infection rate is greater with amniocentesis than CVS.
36. **(D) 70%.** Multiple pregnancies constitute about 3% of all live births. About 70% of twins are dizygotic and 30% are monozygotic. Of the monozygotic twins, one-third (33%) are dichorionic (DC) and two-thirds (67%) are MC.
37. **(C) Absence of a twin-peak sign.** Monochorionic twins are diagnosed by the absence of a twin peak sign (lambda sign) or the presence of

a T-sign where the membranes meet. Similar genders (even in early pregnancy) are not diagnostic of MC twins while a single placenta could be found in DC twins.

38. **(C) From the measurement of CRL of the larger twin.** Where the CRL of multiple pregnancies differ significantly that of the larger twin should be used to date the pregnancies. The head circumference should be used to date the pregnancies if these are >14 weeks gestation.
39. **(C) Preterm delivery.** Complications of twin pregnancies include spontaneous miscarriage, vanishing twin, preterm delivery, eclampsia and preeclampsia, fetal growth restriction, antepartum hemorrhage, anemia, CS, and PPH. The most common complication is preterm delivery which is 6X higher than in singleton pregnancies.
40. **(B) Twin-to-twin transfusion syndrome (TTTS).** The two complications of MC twins that present with polyhydramnios/oligohydramnios sequence are TTTS and TAPS. The bladder is visible in TTTS in stage 1 but with more severe stages stage II and more, this is not visible. In TAPS, the bladder is visible but this is more common after laser treatment for TTTS.
41. **(C) 35–37 weeks.** Timing of delivery in twin pregnancies depends on the type of twins and presence of complications. In the absence of complications, dizygotic twins should be delivered at 37–38 weeks, MC/DA at 35–37 weeks and MC/monoamniotic at 32–34 weeks.
42. **(D) Cephalic/cephalic.** The most common presentation of twins at term is cephalic/cephalic—present in 50% of cases followed by cephalic/breech in 25% of cases. 10% present as breech/cephalic.
43. **(C) If it has not been delivered by 30 minutes.** The delivery of the second twin is said to be delayed if by 30 minutes after delivery of the first it is still to be delivered. Attempts should be made to deliver the second twin within 30 minutes of the first as morbidity and mortality is associated with deliveries occurring after 30 minutes.
44. **(B) 16 weeks.** Ultrasound monitoring for the occurrence of TTTS should start at 16 weeks of gestation. This should be in the form of regular 2 weekly scans for growth, liquor volume, and Doppler of the umbilical and middle cerebral arteries.
45. **(B) If it occurs after 20–24 weeks of gestation.** Bleeding from the genital tract from 20 to 24 weeks of gestation is called antepartum hemorrhage. The precise gestational age at cutoff depends on the country and facilities available for neonatal care.
46. **(B) 5%.** Prior to 24 weeks, placentas that are lying <2 cm from the internal os are classified as low lying. About 95% of these become normally sited by 32 weeks (the so-called placental migration) meaning that only 5% will remain low.

47. **(D) Polyhydramnios.** Risk factors for placenta previa include maternal age >35 years, smoking and cocaine use, multiple pregnancy, high parity, previous CS and previous placenta previa. Polyhydramnios is not a risk factor for placenta previa but for placental abruption.
48. **(D) Placental previa.** The clinical features are classic of placenta previa. The bleeding is painless, occurring in the late second half of pregnancy with no associated fetal compromise. Although local causes could be responsible the fact that this was heavy and is now settling will be in keeping with a major cause of antepartum hemorrhage. Another possible finding would be a high presenting part or an abnormal lie of the fetus.
49. **(E) Ultrasound sound to localize the placenta.** Following a general examination of a patient who presents with mild painless antepartum hemorrhage, an ultrasound scan should be performed to exclude placenta previa. While a FBC is important including securing an IV access, localization of the placenta will influence subsequent management. A speculum and digital examination should be avoided if possible as if the placenta is low lying; this may provoke further significant bleeding.
50. **(D) PPH.** Women with moderate placental abruption are at risk of PPH, usually from a *Couvelaire* uterus. Other complications such as hypovolemic shock, acute renal failure, and DIC are less common except with severe cases.
51. **(C) 34–36 weeks.** Women with diagnosed vasa previa should be delivered at 34–36 weeks so that they do not go into spontaneous labor. If they go into spontaneous labor the vasa previa may rupture and result in significant fetal hemorrhage and mortality or severe morbidity.
52. **(C) 1:10.** Hypertensive disorders of pregnancy are considered one of the most common medical disorders of pregnancy affecting about 1:10 pregnant women.
53. **(E) Urine protein creatinine ratio of >35 µg/mol.** Significant proteinuria is defined as 2+ on urine dipstick or proteinuria of >300 mg/24 hours or protein creatinine ratio of >35 µg/mol.
54. **(E) Interpregnancy interval of at least 120 months.** Prolonged interpregnancy interval defined as at least 10 years is a risk factor for preeclampsia. Other risk factors include maternal age, primiparity, chronic hypertension, medical disorders such as renal disease, diabetes and connective tissue diseases, preeclampsia in previous pregnancy or in first degree relatives, multiple pregnancies, autoimmune disorders, molar pregnancy, and excessive weight gain in pregnancy.
55. **(A) Abnormal trophoblastic invasion of spiral arteries.** Although the etiology of preeclampsia is unknown abnormal trophoblastic

invasion of the spiral arteries leading to ischemia and production of oxidative and inflammatory factors is thought to be involved in the systemic manifestations of preeclampsia.

56. **(B) Hypertension, elevated liver enzymes, and low platelets.** The HELLP syndrome which complicates 2–4% of women with preeclampsia consists of hypertension, elevated liver enzymes, and low platelets. Although proteinuria is a feature in most of these patients it is not required for the diagnosis of HELLP syndrome.
57. **(D) Labetalol.** Labetalol is the drug of first choice for the treatment of hypertension in pregnancy. It can be given orally or intravenously. Other options include alpha-methyldopa and nifedipine. Atenolol is not the treatment of choice in pregnancy as it is associated with an increased risk of fetal growth restriction.
58. **(A) Aspirin from 12 weeks.** Identification of women at high risk of preeclampsia early allows for the institution of measures to reduce the risk of occurrent of preeclampsia. The only known intervention that has been shown to reduce the occurrence of preeclampsia is aspirin from 12 weeks. There are some studies that suggest that calcium supplementation also reduces the risk of hypertensive disorders of pregnancy but current recommendation is the institution of aspirin rather than calcium. The antioxidants vitamin C and E have been shown to cause complications such as fetal growth restriction without reducing the risk of preeclampsia.
59. **(E) ≥10.0%.** Women with preexisting diabetes are advised to optimize their health including good diabetic control before embarking on pregnancy. An ideal HbA1C prior to pregnancy should be <6.5%. If this is 10.0% or more, pregnancy is not advised.
60. **(D) Polyhydramnios.** Complications of poorly controlled diabetes after the late second trimester include macrosomia, IUFD, polyhydramnios, and iatrogenic preterm delivery. Congenital malformations are likely to have been diagnosed early (i.e,. at the time of the anomaly ultrasound scan).
61. **(A) Dietary modification.** Following the diagnosis of gestational diabetes the first approach to management should be dietary modification (the woman should be referred to a dietician) and if this is unsuccessful then and only then should the woman be commenced on metformin and if this fails to control her diabetes she should then be commenced on insulin.
62. **(B) Fasting and 1 or 2 hours postmeals.** Monitoring of diabetes whether Type I, II or gestational in pregnancy is by regular blood glucose measurements including fasting and either 1 or 2 hours postprandial. Type I and II diabetics should in addition have monthly HbA1C measurements.

63. **(B) 37–38^{+6} weeks.** Women with types I or II diabetes that are well controlled should be delivered at 37–38^{+6} weeks or even earlier if the diabetes is poorly controlled.
64. **(D) Around 39–40 weeks.** When gestational diabetes is well controlled the woman can be allowed to deliver at 39–40 weeks and around 37 weeks or even earlier if it is not well controlled.
65. **(A) Congenital malformations.** Complications of thyrotoxicosis in pregnancy include miscarriages, fetal growth restriction, preterm labor, and neonatal thyrotoxicosis [in those with Grave's diseases and thyroid-stimulating hormone (TSH) receptor antibodies]. Congenital malformations and fetal macrosomia are not complications of thyrotoxicosis in pregnancy.
66. **(A) Asymptomatic.** Most women with hypothyroidism in pregnancy are asymptomatic and the diagnosis is based on abnormal thyroid function tests. For those with symptoms, these will include weight gain, intolerance to cold, dry skin, constipation fatigue delayed deep tendon reflexes, and somnolence.
67. **(A) Atopic eruption of pregnancy.** Atopic eruptions of pregnancy (also known as eczema of pregnancy or prurigo gestationis or nurses early-onset prurigo of pregnancy) is characterized by an itching rash that develops around 25–30 weeks. The rash which is typically found on the face, trunk, and extensor surfaces of the limbs is erythematous with excoriations from scratching. Treatment is with emollients, topical antipruritics or steroids, and antihistamines.
68. **(E) Polymorphic eruption of pregnancy (PEP).** Polymorphic eruption of pregnancy also known as pruritic urticarial papules or plaques of pregnancy or toxic erythema of pregnancy present in the third trimester or immediately postpartum with itching and a rash that characteristically spares the periumbilical area. The rash starts on the abdomen and spreads to involve the trunk and extremities but rarely affects the palms and soles. Treatment is with emollients (topical steroids and antihistamines).
69. **(D) Pemphigoid gestationis.** Pemphigoid gestationis also known as pregnancy-induced bullous pemphigoid or gestational pemphigoid or herpes gestationis characteristically presents in the second half of pregnancy with a rash that is typically around the umbilicus and then spreads to the trunk, extremities, and palms and soles but not involving the mucosa. The rash starts as an urticaria that then fuses to form clusters of blisters (bullae) which on clinical examination appear as large and tense blisters mainly around the edges of the rash. Treatment is with a combination of topical or oral corticosteroids and antihistamines.

70. **(B) 5–10%.** Asthma is a common respiratory condition that affects about 5–10% of women in pregnancy.
71. **(E) No impact on the pregnancy.** Well-controlled asthma has no effect on pregnancy; however, poorly controlled asthma can lead to complications including gestational hypertension, fetal growth restriction, and preterm delivery.
72. **(C) A third will remain unchanged.** Pregnancy has variable effects on asthma. About a third will get better, a third will stay the same, and a third will get worse with exacerbations more likely in those with severe asthma than mild asthma. Failure to comply with medications is more common in those who have exacerbations.
73. **(B) Ergometrine.** Women with asthma in pregnancy should be managed as normal but ergometrine and prostaglandin F2α should be avoided as these may cause bronchoconstriction and make the asthma worse.
74. **(B) Lobar pneumonia.** The clinical features are diagnostic of a lobar pneumonia. Bronchial breath sounds are characteristic. In broncho-pneumonia, there are usually widespread crackles (crepitations). Viral infections do not tend to cause such a high temperature and the signs tend to be more generalized if any.
75. **(E) ΔF508.** Cystic fibrosis is an autosomal recessive condition with a carrier frequency of about 1:25 in the general population. The most common nutation which is responsible for about 88% of cases is ΔF508.
76. **(B) Heart block.** The SLE by itself is associated with an increased risk of miscarriages, fetal growth restriction, preeclampsia, VTE, placental abruption, and preterm delivery. These complications are increased irrespective of the presence of anti-Ro/La antibodies. The presence of these antibodies is associated with congenital heart block in about 30% of cases.
77. **(D) Aspirin and low molecular weight heparin.** Antiphospholipid syndrome is associated with complications in pregnancy including recurrent miscarriages. There is some evidence that with a combination of aspirin and low molecular weight heparin, pregnancy outcome is improved in these women.
78. **(D) 42 days (6 weeks).** Thromboprophylaxis should be given for 6 weeks for women with diagnosed connective tissue disease after delivery irrespective of the mode of delivery (cesarean or vaginal).
79. **(E) Heart disease with slight limitation of physical activity.** The NYHA Class I refers to heart disease with no limitation to physical activity while class II refers to associated mild/slight limitation to physical activity and III involves marked limitation and IV inability to carry out any physical activity without discomfort.

80. **(D) Shorten second stage with instrumental delivery and oxytocin for third stage.** For women with cardiac disease in pregnancy that are the NYHA Class II and above the second stage should be shortened with either a ventouse of forceps and the third stage managed with oxytocinon. Syntometrine or ergometrine should be avoided and this increases volume return significantly and may precipitate hypertension and heart failure.
81. **(C) 14 days.** Thromboprophylaxis should be considered antenatally for those with congenital heart disease with pulmonary hypertension or artificial valve replacement or those at risk of atrial fibrillation. Postnatally women with cardiac disease should receive thromboprophylaxis for 14 days.
82. **(D) Infertility treatment.** Risk factors for peripartum cardiomyopathy include ethnicity (African origin), high salt intake, extremes of reproductive age, preeclampsia, malnutrition, and traditional risk factors for cardiovascular disease. Infertility treatment is not a risk factor for cardiomyopathy.
83. **(B) Dilated.** The types of cardiomyopathy include dilated, hypertrophic, arrhythmogenic, right ventricular, restrictive, Takotsubo, and left ventricular noncompaction. Of these, the dilated and hypertrophic types are the most common.
84. **(C) Marfan syndrome.** Marfan syndrome is the cardiac condition which is inherited as an autosomal dominant condition with a mortality as high as up to 50% in those with marked aortic dilatation.
85. **(B) Affects 2–10% of women.** Asymptomatic bacteriuria affects 2–10% of pregnant women—a prevalence similar to that in nonpregnant women.
86. **(D) 30%.** Untreated, 30% of those with asymptomatic bacteriuria will progress to acute pyelonephritis. At least 1% of pregnant women have one episode of acute pyelonephritis in pregnancy.
87. **(A) *Escherichia coli.*** *E. coli* is the most common cause of urinary tract infection in pregnancy. As a gram-negative organism, if untreated, can progress to gram-negative septicemia—an important cause of maternal morbidity and mortality.
88. **(C) 12–24 months.** Ideally women should wait for 1–2 years after a renal transplant before embarking on pregnancy. However, if after 6 months there is no evidence of rejection, renal function is stable and the patient is on minimal immunosuppressants, then pregnancy could be considered.
89. **(A) BP, medications, renal function (creatinine), and proteinuria.** At the prepregnancy clinic, it is important to ensure that the graft is stable, and creatinine is <1.4 mg/kg/dL, BP is <140/90 mm Hg,

proteinuria is <500 mg/24 hours and all drugs contraindicated in pregnancy [e.g., angiotensin-converting enzyme inhibitor (ACEi), mycophenolate mofetil, and tacrolimus] are stopped/changed.

90. **(B) CMV.** Microcephaly as a congenital malformation is associated with infections which include CMV, rubella, toxoplasmosis, and Zika virus. Parvovirus B19 is associated with fetal anemia and hydrops while vertical transmission is rare with the coronaviruses.
91. **(E) Varicella zoster.** Infections with varicella zoster and toxoplasmosis are known induce a lifelong immunity. While previous infections with herpes and CMV may modify the course of subsequent infections, they do not confer lifelong immunity.
92. **(A) CMV.** The CMV is the most common viral infection in pregnancy.
93. **(C) 48 hours before the rash and until it has crusted.** Anyone with chickenpox is infectious 48 hours before the rash appears and until it crusts (which is usually 5 days). Significant contact defined as being in the same room for at least 15 minutes is required for transmission to occur.
94. **(C) Parvovirus B19.** The most common cause of nonimmune hydrops is infection with parvovirus B19. Although some of the other infections can cause hydrops infections, parvovirus B19 is considered the most common.
95. **(C) Fluid from blisters for viral PCR and then screen for other sexually transmitted infections (STIs).** The diagnosis of herpes simplex infection is best by PCR of fluid from vesicles or swabs from herpetic ulcers. Screening for other STIs should be offered to women with genital herpes (including *Chlamydia trachomatis, Neisseria gonorrhoeae,* HIV, and hepatitis B).
96. **(D) HBV e antigen positive, and e antibody negative.** The highest risk of vertical transmission is in women who are HBV e antigen positive and antibody negative. About 85% of neonates born to mothers who are e antigen positive will become early carriers and subsequently become chronic carriers.
97. **(A) <50 ribonucleic acid (RNA) copies/mL.** The aim of antiretroviral therapy (ART) for HIV positive women in pregnancy is to ensure that the viral load is at its lowest from about 36 weeks to allow for a vaginal delivery with the lowest risk of vertical transmission (>80% of vertical transmission occurs after 36 weeks and intrapartum). The threshold viral load is <50 RNA copies/mL.
98. **(A) Coronavirus disease-2019 (COVID-19).** The SARS-CoV-2 causes the disease COVID-19. It started in December 2019 in Wuhan province China and was declared a pandemic by the World Health Organization (WHO) in March 2020.

99. **(A) In the first trimester.** Infections such as toxoplasmosis that cause congenital malformations in pregnancy pose the greatest risk to the fetus if they occur in the first trimester. The highest vertical transmission (with *T. gondii*); however, occurs with infection in the third trimester but this does not have severe consequences on the fetus.
100. **(D) Toxoplasmosis.** Toxoplasmosis is a protozoal infection that is transmitted by ingesting food (vegetables or beef) with oocytes of contaminated water. Cat litters are also a source of the infection.
101. **(D) Treponema pallidum hemagglutination assay (TPHA).** In the screening for syphilis in pregnancy the first tests that are usually offered are the nontreponemal test and these are either VDRL or RPR test. If any of these are positive then the treponemal test would have to be performed and these include the TPHA or fluorescent treponemal antibody absorption (FTA-ABS). There is no place for PCR or culture unless there are lesions from which samples can be obtained.
102. **(E) Streptomycin.** Among the drugs used to treat pulmonary tuberculosis, streptomycin is contraindicated in pregnancy. It is associated with the 8th cranial nerve damage. The others can be used if indicated.
103. **(A) *Chlamydia trachomatis*.** Sticky eyes that develop within a few days of delivery are indicative of infections acquired during birth. If the symptoms develop within 2–4 days the cause is usually gonococcal but if these develop between 5 and 14 days *Chlamydia trachomatis* is the usual cause.
104. **(A) By attacking the erythroid progenitor cells leading to anemic heart failure.** Parvovirus is the most common cause of nonimmune hydrops. This is through attacking fetal erythroid progenitor cells shortening their lifespan with resultant anemia and anemic heart failure.
105. **(E) Aciclovir from now until delivery by elective CS at 39 weeks.** When primary genital herpes is diagnosed from 36 weeks of gestation, suppressive aciclovir 400 mg tds should be administered until delivery by CS (primary infection within 6 weeks of delivery is an indication for CS).
106. **(D) IM crystalline penicillin.** The treatment of choice for syphilis irrespective of the stage is IM crystalline penicillin (Penicillin G or Benzathine penicillin). It is not an indication for termination of pregnancy although untreated; there is an increased risk of congenital malformations.
107. **(A) Ampicillin.** The treatment of choice for listeriosis is parenteral ampicillin 2 g every 6 hours. If there is allergy to penicillin then the combination of trimethoprim and sulfamethoxazole can be used.

108.

	HSV1 immunoglobulin M (IgM)	HSV2 IgM	HSV1 immunoglobulin G (IgG)	HSV2 IgG
D	Absent	Present	Present	Absent

Genital herpes can either be primary, recurrent, or nonprimary first episode. This is based on serology. In primary infections there are no IgG antibodies to the subtype of herpes while in recurrent episodes there are IgG antibodies to the subtype. Nonprimary episodes are infections of a different subtype in a patient who has previously been infected with the other subtype, i.e., there are IgG antibodies to the other subtype.

109. **(C) Previous postpartum depression.** With regards to risk factors for postpartum depression the recurrence is highest with a history of severe depression, especially if it was in a previous pregnancy. The recurrence risk 50%.

110. **(C) 10–15%.** Severe postpartum depression affects about 10–15% of women after within 12 months of childbirth.

111. **(B) Postpartum blues.** Postpartum blues are experienced by up to 80% of women within 2–3 days postpartum. They typically present with mood swings, crying spells, anxiety, difficulties sleeping, lack of energy, feeling overwhelmed, reduced concentration, irritability, and poor appetite. These are not associated with negative feelings toward the baby or self-harm. The symptoms tend to be self-limiting and resolve within 1–2 weeks.

112. **(A) Hemorrhage.** Causes of maternal collapse in pregnancy (or indeed in a person) can be grouped under 4Hs (hypovolemia, hypothermia, hypokalemia or hyponatremia, and hypoxia) and 4Ts (thromboembolism, toxicity, tamponade, and tension pneumothorax). The most common cause in pregnancy is hypovolemia from hemorrhage.

113. **(A) Blood culture and lactate and initiation of broad-spectrum antibiotics covering gram-negative, positive, and anaerobes.** In the management of sepsis, the most important step consists of obtaining blood cultures, quantification of serum lactate, and initiation of IV antibiotic therapy. The antibiotics must cover gram-negative and positive organisms as well as anaerobes. Serum lactate will help determine the severity of sepsis. A value of 4 or more mmol/L is indicative of severe sepsis.

114. **(A) 1:1,000 IM.** Adrenaline for the treatment of anaphylaxis should be administered either intramuscularly (IM) or intravenously (IV). The IM dose is 1:1000 (0.5 mL) while the IV dose is 1:10,000 (0.5 mL).

115. **(C) 24 weeks.** An IUFD is considered late if it occurs from 24 weeks of gestation. In the low-income countries the gestational age may be increased to 28 weeks while in some of the high-income countries it may be lowered to 20 weeks. In general, however, 24 weeks is considered the current cut-off gestation.
116. **(C) Absence of fetal heart motion on 2D ultrasound.** The confirmation of an IUFD is best with a 2D ultrasound scan demonstrating absent fetal heart movements and maybe Spalding depending on the time of death. Color flow Doppler would further improve the accuracy of diagnosis.
117. **(C) To help provide answers and plan care in the next pregnancy.** Investigating for an intrauterine death is important primarily to provide answers to why (if these can be found) and plan management of subsequent pregnancies (i.e., what the recurrence rate is and how this can be prevented). Although the results help parents come to terms with the loss and indeed plan management these are not the primary reasons for investigating.
118. **(A) All women irrespective of their blood group.** Kleihauer test is performed to check for lethal fetomaternal hemorrhage. It should be performed on all women with an IUFD and not simply on those who are rhesus negative. It should be undertaken before birth as red cells might clear quickly from the maternal circulation.
119. **(B) 24–28 weeks.** Preterm labor is defined as onset of labor before 37 completed weeks. It is very preterm if its labor between 24 and 28 weeks, early preterm if between 28 and 34 weeks and later preterm between 34 and 37 weeks.
120. **(D) Increased 4.9-fold.** Previous preterm delivery is the strongest predictor of another preterm birth. The risk increases 2.2-fold after one, 3.7-fold after 2, and 4.9-fold after 3.
121. **(C) Previous preterm delivery.** Risk factors for preterm delivery include age (higher in older and younger mothers, especially those having their first babies), previous preterm delivery, prelabor rupture of membranes, sociodemographic factors (smoking, alcohol, use of recreational drugs, and poor nutrition), infections, multiple pregnancies, cervical weakness, medical disorders especially preeclampsia, diabetes mellitus, malformations of the uterus, polyhydramnios, and maternal stress. Of all of these, the strongest predictor is previous preterm birth with the risk more than doubling after one, increasing to 3.7-fold after 2 and to 4.9-fold after 3.
122. **(A) <25 mm.** With regards to cervical assessment at 22 weeks the length and appearance of the cervix are used in classifying women into high or low risk. A cervical length of <25 mm or funneling is associated with a significantly high risk of preterm delivery.

123. **(C) 14–16 weeks.** Women with suspected cervical weakness should have serial cervical assessment from 14 weeks and a cerclage inserted when the cervix is shortening or funneling is occurring. Where a decision has been taken to insert a cerclage on the basis of history this should be inserted between 14 and 16 weeks.
124. **(C) CBC, urinalysis, corticosteroids, and commence on tocolysis with nifedipine.** Women presenting with preterm contractions should be assessed (general examination and cervical assessment) and investigation (urinalysis, CBC, and swabs if indicated) and corticosteroids administered and tocolysis commenced. The tocolytic of choice is nifedipine—it is as effective as atosiban (the calcium channel blocker) but is cheaper, easier to administer and has fewer side effects.
125. **(B) She is 24–32 weeks.** Magnesium sulfate should be given for neuroprotection to women presenting in preterm labor between 24 and 32 weeks. The benefit of this before 24 weeks is questionable.
126. **(E) Speculum examination.** Confirmation of rupture of fetal membranes is mainly by speculum examination but where there is doubt (i.e., there is no obvious fluid coming through the cervix or in the vagina, the Partus™ test is recommended). Tests such as the nitrazine paper test and ferning are very rarely used in contemporary obstetrics.
127. **(B) Hb <110 g/L in the first half and <105 g/L in the second half of pregnancy.** Anemia in pregnancy is defined as Hb <110 g/L in the first half and <105 g/L in the second half. The hemodilution effect of increased plasma volume is responsible for the change in definition in the second half of pregnancy.
128. **(D) Iron deficiency.** Iron deficiency is the most common type of anemia. It could be as result of reduced intake or malabsorption.
129. **(D) 2:4.** The risk of the couple has a child with HbAA or sickle cell is 1:4 and that of having a carrier is 2:4 (50%)
130. **(E) Transfusion of at least 8 times per year.** Categorization of beta-thalassemia into major or intermedia is based on the number of blood transfusions received per year. Transfusion for at least eight times per years is considered major while less is intermedia.
131. **(B) Heart.** Thalassemia major results in high iron load which may affect multiple systems. It particularly affects the heart causing a cardiomyopathy. It is therefore important that women who are planning pregnancy should have an echo as well and chelating to reduce the iron load.
132. **(D) None-invasive diagnosis (NIPD).** Prenatal diagnosis of single gene defects such as hemoglobinopathies, blood groups, and CF can now be made from circulating free fetal deoxyribonucleic acid (DNA).

The test for this is NIPD which is performed from 9 weeks of gestation. It has an advantage that it is not associated with any risk to the fetus.

133. **(A) 6–10 days.** Postpartum thromboprophylaxis with low molecular weight heparin is recommended for 6–10 days for women with sickle cell anemia or SCD after a vaginal delivery but this should be extended for 6 weeks (42 days) if delivery is by CS.
134. **(B) At booking and at 28 weeks.** Blood group, Rhesus type, and atypical antibodies should be checked at booking and then again at 28 weeks.
135. **(D) 250 IU.** For sensitizing events before 20 weeks 250 IU of anti-D should be administered and after 20 weeks this should be 500 IU. This covers up to 4 mL of fetal blood in the maternal circulation.
136. **(B) Cord blood for genotype and if positive check Kleihauer and administer 500 IU anti-D within 72 hours.** The woman is at risk of sensitization after delivery; however, if her baby is Rhesus (D) negative she will not require anti-D. Cord blood for fetal Rhesus type should be collected at birth and if it is positive maternal Kleihauer should be checked but this should not delay administration of anti-D. The Kleihauer test is just to ensure that the administered anti-D is enough to cover any fetomaternal hemorrhage.
137. **(D) Protein S.** Clotting factors which rise in pregnancy include factors VII, VIII, IX, and XI while others remain unchanged but protein S levels fall.
138. **(D) Increased 6–12 fold.** Pregnancy increases the risk of VTE 6–12 fold. This risk is greater after a CS than a vaginal delivery.
139. **(D) From 0 to 2 weeks postpartum.** The risk of VTE is greatest in the first 2 weeks postpartum but VTE can occur at any stage in pregnancy including the first trimester.
140. **(C) Degenerating fibroid.** Degenerating fibroids are a common cause of abdominal pain in pregnancy. They typically present with localized constant pain which is nonradiating and not associated with systemic symptoms. Clinically the pain is localized and the uterus may be larger than dates. Because fibroids become softer in pregnancy it may be difficult to palpate them. In this patient a history of heavy periods and the nature of the pain and findings on examination point to the diagnosis.
141. **(A) Acute appendicitis.** Acute appendicitis is the most common cause of surgical pain in the abdomen in pregnancy. It commonly occurs in the second trimester as in this patient and classically presents with pain that is central and then shifts to the right lower abdomen. It may be associated with systemic symptoms such as nausea, vomiting, and fever as in this patient. Ultrasound scan maybe helpful in diagnosis and treatment is surgical.

142. **(A) Contracted pelvis.** There are several reasons for induction of labor (fetal and maternal) and few contraindications including two or more previous CS, severe fetal compromise (where the fetus will not withstand the stress of labor), abnormal lie of the fetus (transverse or oblique), and a contracted pelvis.
143. **(C) 6.** A Bishop's score >6 is considered favorable for induction of labor and is associated with a short induction-delivery interval.
144. **(A) Attitude of the fetal presenting part.** Constituents of the Bishop's score include position of the cervix (anterior, mid, or posterior) consistency (firm, medium, or soft), length/effacement (>2 cm, 1–2 cm, 0.5–1 cm, or <0.5 cm), dilation (0–2, 3–4, and >4), and station (0–3, 0–2, and 0–1 and 0+).
145. **(D) Prostaglandin E2 given as vaginal tablets or gel followed by artificial rupture of membranes with or without oxytocinon.** Induction of labor can be performed medically, surgically, mechanically, or a combination. The most common approach is a combination of prostaglandin vaginal tablets or pessaries followed by artificial rupture of membranes and IV oxytocinon if contractions are not initiated.
146. **(D) Ruptured uterus.** Induction of labor may be followed by complications which are fetal or maternal. Maternal complications include uterine hyperstimulation (tachysystole), uterine rupture, fluid overload, failed induction, and PPH while fetal complications include cord prolapse, fetal distress from tachysystole, and neonatal jaundice if oxytocinon is used. Uterine rupture is more common in multiparous women or those who have had surgery on the uterus (myomectomy or previous CS) and typically present with sudden onset abdominal pain or maternal collapse and fetal bradycardia as in this patient. Fetal parts are easy to palpate abdominally and the presenting part might recede.
147. **(C) 11.0 cm.** At the pelvic inlet, the transverse diameter is larger than the anteroposterior (AP) (13.5 cm versus 11.0 cm), in the mid cavity these are same (12.0 cm) while at the outlet the AP diameter is larger than the inlet (13.5 cm versus 11.0 cm) i.e., the reverse at the inlet.
148. **(E) Scaphoid.** The four types of pelvises are gynecoid (the most common), android, anthropoid, and platypelloid). Scaphoid is not a type of pelvis.
149. **(B) Frontal and parietal to form the sagittal suture.** The four sutures of the fetal skull are the frontal formed by the frontal bones, the sagittal formed by the parietal bones, the coronal between the frontal and parietal bones, and the lambdoidal formed by the occipital and the parietal bones.
150. **(A) Left occipito-anterior.** The position of the presenting part is defined based on the relationship of the occiput with the pelvis.

Occipito-anterior, lateral, or posterior if it is anterior, lateral, or posterior. If the lie is oblique (i.e., the fontanelles are between 12 and 3 or between 3 and 6 o'clock positions these are described as right or left occipito anterior or posterior respectively and when the occiput is at 3 or 9 o'clock positions it is said to be occipito-transverse.

151. **(B) Occipito-mental.** The diameter at the pelvic inlet is suboccipito-bregmatic for a well-flexed vertex presentation, occipito-frontal for a deflexed (occipito-frontal), occipito-mental for brow presentation, and suboccipito-bregmatic for face presentation.
152. **(A) Of origin in the uterine fundus and spreading downward.** Normal uterine contractions originate from the uterine fundus and spread downward. When these originate from the lower uterus and spread upward they are described as abnormal.
153. **(D) When they occur at a frequency of 3–4 in 10 minutes with each lasting 30–45 seconds.** Contractions are defined as normal when they occur at a frequency of 3–4 in 10 minutes and each lasting about 30–45 seconds. When the contractions are too frequent (>5/10 minutes) tachysystole is a considered diagnosis and infrequent contractions are associated with poor progress in labor.
154. **(D) The maximum diameter of the presenting part has entered the pelvic brim.** Engagement is defined as the time when the maximum diameter of the presenting part has entered the pelvic brim (i.e., at least three-fifths of the head is in the pelvis). Clinically this is diagnosed when at most two-fifths of the head can be palpated abdominally. A fixed head is not the same as an engaged head.
155. **(E) Reassessment at 4 hours.** For women in normal labor the acceptable contraction rate is three to four in 10 minutes with each contraction lasting about 30–60 minutes. Progress of labor is however the most important marker for efficient uterine contractions and this is measured by cervical dilatation and descent of the presenting part. Dilatation is normal if it occurs at a rate of at least 0.5 cm/hour. In this patient, a dilation of 2 cm over 4 hours is acceptable and therefore the plan should be to review her after 4 hours. There is no need to interfere to accelerate labor.
156. **(A) <7.21.** A fetal blood sample pH of at least 7.25 is considered normal (and implying that the next sampling could be done after 1 hour) while a value between 7.21 and 7.24 is considered a borderline result requiring repeating within 30 minutes and a value below 7.21 is indicative of delivery.
157. **(C) <–7 mEq/L.** The normal base excess from a fetal blood sample is –7 mEq/L to –4 mEq/L. Values above –4 mEq/L are indicative of acidosis.

158. **(D) Pushing for >120 minutes.** The active second stage of labor defined as the start of time of urge to push (pushing) to delivery is 2 hours in a primigravida and 1 hour in a multiparous woman. The duration of the passive second stage in a primigravida with an epidural is 2 hours. An active second stage that is longer than 120 minutes in a primigravida is therefore considered prolonged.

159. **(D) 60 minutes.** The placenta in most women should be delivered within 4–5 minutes of delivery of the baby and the duration of the third stage should not be >30 minutes. For patients who opt for physiological management of the third stage this should be abandoned and active management instituted if the placenta has not been delivered after 60 minutes.

160. **(B) Blood loss of at least 500 mL within 24 hours of delivery.** Primary PPH is defined as bleeding in excess of 500 mL within the first 24 hours of birth. This may be lower depending on the starting Hb of the woman. Bleeding after 24 hours is secondary PPH.

161. **(D) Oxygen saturation.** Components of APGAR score include appearance, pulse rate, grimace, activity, and respiratory effort. The total score is out of 10 and the score is commonly done at 1 and 5 minutes. The 5-minute score is a better reflection of the fetal state compared to the 1-minute score. A score of 8 or above is considered as normal while a score of <6 is considered abnormal and 6–7 borderline.

162. **(E) Increased risk of neonatal respiratory depression.** The disadvantages of administering opioid analgesia to the mother close to delivery are mainly that of neonatal depression. This can be reversed with naloxone. The mother is also at an increased risk of nausea, vomiting, drowsiness, sedation, and delayed gastric emptying which may be complicated by aspiration especially with general anesthesia (GA). While the maternal risks are important these are rare but the neonatal respiratory depression is the most significant.

163. **(D) Obstetrics cholestasis.** With regards to opioids in labor, diamorphine is preferred over pethidine. Pethidine is not recommended for women who have SCD, obstetrics cholestasis, and anemia.

164. **(C) Dysfunctional uterine contractions.** The most common cause of labor dystocia (poor progress in labor) is abnormal uterine activity (dysfunctional uterine contractions) from several factors including dehydration and acidosis/ketosis. Other causes include abnormal presentation and position and cephalopelvic disproportion.

165. **(E) Tight fitting head with cervical edema.** When there is obstructive labor, clinical features include a tight fitting head with or without cervical edema, caput +++, and moulding +++. Although a high head may be suggestive of disproportion it is not a diagnostic feature.

166. **(D) Suboccipito-bregmatic.** The presenting diameter in face presentation is suboccipito-bregmatic which is about 9.5 cm. Face presentation with the chin anterior (mentoanterior) can be allowed to deliver vaginally but mentoposterior positions are unlikely to be delivered successfully vaginally and these are best delivered by CS.
167. **(C) Labor lasting <2 hours.** Precipitate labor is defined as labor whose duration is <2 hours. It is associated with fetal and maternal complications including trauma (fetal and maternal) and PPH.
168. **(C) The shoulders have not been delivered after 60 seconds from delivery of the head.** Shoulder dystocia is a complication in which the shoulders of the baby are obstructed and need additional maneuvers to be delivered. The diagnosis is made if the shoulders have not been delivered after 60 seconds from the delivery of the head.
169. **(D) Failure to deliver it within 60 minutes of delivery of the baby if physiological management of the third stage.** The placenta is said to be retained if it has not been delivered within 30 minutes or 60 minutes of active or physiological management of the third stage of labor, respectively.
170. **(C) Maternal age >35 years.** Risk factors for shoulder dystocia include previous shoulder dystocia (associated with a recurrent risk of 10%), fetal macrosomia, diabetes mellitus, maternal obesity, and induction of labor. Maternal age is not a risk factor for shoulder dystocia.
171. **(B) 32 weeks.** The incidence of breech presentation at term is 2–4% but at 28 weeks of gestation, this is about 20%. This rises to 25% at 32 weeks and then gradually falls to 24% at term.
172. **(D) 37–38 weeks.** In uncomplicated pregnancies, ECV for breech presentations should be offered at 37–38 weeks. About 50–60% of these will be successful.
173. **(C) Idiopathic.** Although there are risk factors for breech presentation, in most cases none of these risks are present and the breech is therefore considered idiopathic.
174. **(D) Preterm <34 weeks.** Contraindications to instrumental deliveries include preterm <34 weeks, babies with bleeding or suspected bleeding disorders, breech, or face presentation. Caution should be exercised when performing an instrumental delivery in the presence of vulva varicosities but these are no considered a contraindication.
175. **(D) The flexion point.** In placing the ventouse it is important to examine the vertex to determine the flexion point on the fetal head. This is defined as 6 cm from the anterior fontanelle and 3 cm from the posterior fontanelle. The cup should be placed over this point.
176. **(C) Failure to deliver the head after three pulls.** A failed instrumental delivery is defined as one in which following successful application

the head of the baby is not delivered after three pulls. The use of sequential instruments (ventouse followed by forceps) is discouraged and this is only allowed if delivery with a forceps is considered very easy (i.e., the head is sitting on the perineum).

177. **(D) 12 hours.** Following an instrumental delivery, it is recommended that if this is performed under regional anesthesia, a catheter should be left in situ for 12 hours as there is an increased risk of bladder dysfunction. Following removal of the catheter, residual volume should be measured after voiding.
178. **(C) 70%.** The success rate of VBAC is usually about 70%. This much higher is if the CS was on a woman who has already had a normal vaginal delivery.
179. **(B) 0.5% (1:200).** The risk of uterine rupture in labor following a previous lower segment CS is estimated to be 1:200 (0.5%). This risk rises with the number of CS hence the usual recommendation is that after two CS, delivery should best be by a repeat CS.
180. **(E) Increased risk of transient tachypnea of the newborn (TTN).** Complications of elective CS include maternal hemorrhage, visceral injuries, cesarean hysterectomy, injury to the baby, and increased placental previa in subsequent pregnancies. The timing of delivery is important as delivery before 39 weeks is associated with an increased risk of TTN.
181. **(C) Third degree category A.** A perineal tear is defined as injury to the perineum which is categorized into first, second, third, and fourth degrees. A third-degree tear involves the perineum and anal sphincter muscles but not the mucosa. This is further categorized in A, B, or C with involvement of <50% of the external sphincter known as category A, involvement of >50% of the external anal sphincter is category B and involvement of both the internal and external sphincters category C. When the rectal mucosa is involved it is a fourth-degree tear.
182. **(D) All third- and fourth-degree perineal tears.** Following the repair of third- and fourth-degree perineal tears, the patient should be placed on antibiotics for about 5–7 days and also given stool softeners such as lactulose.
183. **(D) Blood loss of >2,000 mL.** Primary PPH between 500 and 1,000 mL is classified as minor PPH while any loss above 1,000 mL is major PPH. Loss of between 1,000 and 2,000 mL is moderate major PPH and above 2,000 mL is severe major PPH.
184. **(C) 10–15%.** Primary PPH affects 10–15% of deliveries and is an important cause of maternal morbidity and mortality worldwide.
185. **(D) Uterine atony.** Several risk factors increase the risk of primary PPH. These include uterine overdistension conditions, uterine fibroids, bleeding disorders, maternal obesity, macrosomia, placenta previa,

previous PPH, prolonged labor, syntocinon augmentation, retained placenta, instrumental delivery, placental abruption, uterine rupture, antepartum hemorrhage, and cervical, vaginal, or perineal tears. A large number of these result in uterine atony which is the most common cause of primary PPH.

186. **(D) Rub uterine contractions while asking for completeness of the placenta and membranes.** The first step to take in the management of mild primary PPH (especially minor PPH) is to rub uterine contractions while at the same time asking about the completeness of the placenta and membranes. Once this has been achieved, the bladder should be emptied and the uterus and vagina evacuated of blood clots. Subsequent management will depend on findings and response of the uterus to massaging.
187. **(A) A total of eight 0.25 micrograms doses.** In the algorithm of managing primary PPH, when a decision is taken to administer carboprost, it should be given as eight doses of 0.25 micrograms every 15 minutes.
188. **(C) Prostaglandin induction of labor.** The risk of uterine rupture in women who have had one previous CS that labor spontaneously is 0.5% (1:200). The use of prostaglandins increases this risk significantly by about 3–4 folds. Although the use of syntocinon is associated with an increased risk this is not as high as with prostaglandins.
189. **(E) Well-contracted uterus.** Uterine inversion is a cause of PPH and collapse. The clinical features are typically not in consonant with the degree of hemorrhage as the collapse may be related to vasovagal attack. Clinically the uterus is hypotonic with a dimple in the fundus and maybe a mass in the vaginal depending on the stage of the inversion.
190. **(D) 10–14 days.** Following delivery of the placenta the uterus starts contracting and retracting (involution). It becomes a pelvic organ (i.e., not palpable per abdomen) after 10–14 days.
191. **(C) 4–7.** Blood-stained discharge after birth which consists of necrotic decidua and blood is known as lochia. Its color is red to start with and this is known as *Lochia rubra* and changes to pink (*Lochia serosa*) toward the end of the first week and toward the end of the week this changes to a yellowish-whitish discharge (*Lochia alba*) which may last up to a month.
192. **(C) 3 weeks after delivery.** Ovulation resumes by the end of the third week if the woman is not breastfeeding. In most nonbreastfeeding mothers, periods would have resumed within 4–6 weeks postpartum.
193. **(E) 80%.** Approximately 80% of women experience perineal pain in the first 3–10 days after a vaginal delivery. Nearly all women who have had an instrumental delivery will experience perineal pain.

194. **(D) 6 weeks.** Abdominal stretch exercises are encouraged after delivery. These should be started about 2 weeks after a vaginal delivery and 6 weeks after a CS.
195. **(D) A temperature of at least 38°C on more than two occasions after 24 hours of delivery and up to 14 days.** Puerperal pyrexia is defined as a temperature of 38°C or more on more than two occasions after 24 hours of delivery and up to 14 days postpartum.
196. **(B) *Escherichia coli.*** Of the organisms that cause puerperal pyrexia, *Escherichia coli* is the most common and it causes gram-negative infections that may cause sepsis.
197. **(C) Blood cultures and prompt administration of IV antibiotic covering gram-negative and positive organisms and anaerobes.** The first and most important step to take in the management of sepsis according to the "Surviving Sepsis" guidelines is blood cultures and prompt IV administration of antibiotics covering gram-negative and positive and anaerobic organisms. Although other investigations such as urea and electrolytes, blood lactate, FBC, arterial blood gases, and markers of sepsis are important, these must not take priority over initiation of antibiotics. Blood cultures should be obtained before antibiotics as this allows for identification of the organisms involved and their sensitivity profile.
198. **(A) *Clostridium perfringens.*** Infection with *Clostridium perfringens* which causes gas gangrene is likely to cause tissue necrosis and treatment may require excision/debridement of the necrotic tissue for this to be effective.
199. **(B) >4 mmol/L.** Where available serum lactate is useful in categorizing sepsis. It is severe if the levels are >4 mmol/L.
200. **(A) From second to third day postpartum.** Colostrum is the yellowish fluid produced by the breast from as early as the sixteenth week of pregnancy and is replaced by milk from the second to the third day postpartum.
201. **(D) Cow's milk contains more protein.** Human milk contains more fat and lactulose but less protein and sodium. The caloric content of human milk is 75 kcal/mL compared to 66 kcal/mL for cow's milk. The water content of both is about the same.
202. **(C) Provides more immunoglobulins.** Colostrum which is produced from as early as the 16th week of pregnancy provides the baby with immunoglobulins more than human and cow's milk and this serves as protection against infections. It contains more protein than both human and cow's milk but less fat and lactose.
203. **(A) Increase risk of juvenile diabetes.** Breastfeeding has several advantages over bottle feeding. Some of these include the fact that it is cheaper and natural, provides a natural balance of nutrients for

the baby including immunoglobulins, is associated with a lower risk of atopic conditions (eczema and asthma), necrotizing enterocolitis in premature and severely growth restricted babies, childhood gastroenteritis, and juvenile diabetes.

204. **(B) Avoid expression, analgesics, and firm bra for 2 weeks.** For those who do not wish to breastfeed or have a reason for lactation suppression, the first approach is to recommend avoiding expression, simple analgesics (like acetaminophen) and a firm bra for 2 weeks. If this is unsuccessful then dopamine agonist such as bromocriptine and cabergoline can be recommended. With these agents, ovulation returns quickly hence the women must be counseled properly about pregnancy.
205. **(D) Flucloxacillin and acetaminophen.** The treatment of choice for mastitis is a broad-spectrum antibiotic and an anti-inflammatory agent. The antibiotic of choice is flucloxacillin.
206. **(C) The total number of stillbirths and early neonatal deaths per 1,000 total births.** Perinatal mortality rate is defined as the total number of stillbirths (delivery of a baby without signs of life after 24 weeks) and early neonatal death (death in the first week of life irrespective of gestation at delivery) per 1,000 total births (still and live births).
207. **(E) Unexplained.** About a quarter of stillbirths are unexplained in high-income countries. The next most common causes of stillbirths are antepartum and intrapartum hemorrhage (12.9%), intrauterine growth restriction (10.2%), placental abnormalities/pathology (9.3%), and congenital malformations (9.1%).
208. **(B) Hemorrhage.** Hemorrhage is the most common direct cause of maternal death worldwide. In the UK, VTE is the most common direct cause.
209. **(B) 6 weeks.** Maternal mortality is defined as death of the mother during pregnancy, childbirth, and up to 42 days (6 weeks) after delivery. In the UK death between 43 days and 12 months is classified as late maternal death.
210. **(A) Type 1.** Type 1 FGM involves partial or total removal of the clitoris (clitoridectomy) as in this patient.
211. **(B) Narrowing of the vaginal orifice with the creation of a covering seal by cutting and appositioning the labia minora.** In Type 2 FGM, there is partial or total removal of the clitoris and labia minor with or without excision of the labia majora (excision) whereas in type 3 there is narrowing of the vaginal orifice by creating a covering seal from cutting and bringing together the labia majora. All other types of harmful procedure including piercing, scratching, scarring, and diathermy are classed as type 4.

212. **(D) Around 20 weeks.** Women booking for antenatal care who have had FGM should have an examination of the vulva to determine whether de-infibulation is indicated. Where the introitus is so narrow as not to permit urination or examination, consideration should be given to de-infibulation. It is recommended that this is either done around 20 weeks or in labor (first stage) or at the time of delivery or postoperatively after a CS.

213. **(E) Preterm delivery.** Complications of FGM can be immediate or long-term. Complications unique to pregnancy include anxiety, PTSD, prolonged labor, difficulties performing a vaginal examination, perineal trauma, PPH, increased risk of CS, stillbirth and neonatal death, and obstetric fistula formation. Preterm delivery is not a known complication of FGM.

214. **(E) Preterm delivery.** There is no evidence that fasting in the first and third trimesters (by women who maintain a balanced diet) has a detrimental effect on the pregnancy (i.e., there are no data to suggest an increase in risk of complications). Fasting in the second trimester (from 22 to 27 weeks) when fetal growth is maximum has however been shown to be associated with an increased risk of preterm delivery.

215. **(E) Spontaneous preterm labor.** The main risks of fasting in women with diabetes include hypoglycemia, hyperglycemia, ketoacidosis, difficulties with glycemic control, and various fetal complications depending on how these complications are management. Although preterm delivery is slightly higher it is iatrogenic rather than spontaneous.

216. **(E) Sweating and chills.** It is important that when pregnant women who are diabetic and are fasting present as emergency with features of poor glycemic control, hypoglycemia must be distinguished from hyperglycemia as management of the two is different. Hypoglycemia will present with trembling, sweating/shills, palpitations hunger, altered mental state, confusion, and headaches while hyperglycemia will present with nausea/vomiting, abdominal pain, extreme thirst, hunger, frequent micturition, fatigue (tiredness), and confusion. In this patient, a clinical feature that will confirm the diagnosis of hypoglycemia will therefore be those features unique to hypoglycemia and these include trembling, sweating/chills, and palpitations.

217. **(F) 25% will be normal, 25% affected, and 50% will be carriers.** Cystic fibrosis is an autosomal recessive condition. For autosomal recessive conditions, transmission is horizontal (normal parents often have more than one affected child). Carrier parents have a 50% chance of having a carrier and a 25% chance of having an affected or a normal child.

218. **(E) 50% of males are affected and 50% of females are carriers.** For sex-linked recessive disorders like hemophilia A, none of the female offspring will be affected. The condition is usually transmitted by asymptomatic females hence for the carrier mother, 50% of her sons will be affected and 50% of her daughters will be carriers. If the father has the condition then none of his sons will be affected but all his daughters will be carriers.

219. **(D) Sex-determining region on Y chromosome.** Germ cells migrate from the yolk sac to the lie underneath the epithelium of the genital ridge and are undifferentiated up to 7 weeks. Thereafter, in males the presence of the SRY-region on the Y chromosome causes these to differentiate into testes. In its absence, the gonads develop into ovaries.

220. **(A) Absence of AMH.** The absence of AMH allows the Müllerian ducts to grow downward and medially fusing in their lower part to form the fallopian tubes, uterus, cervix, and the upper two-thirds of the vagina.

Index

A

Abdomen, magnetic resonance imaging of 36
Acetaminophen 220
Acetic acid 76
Aciclovir 32, 105, 142, 208
Acne 99
Acupuncture 21
Adenocarcinoma 34, 77
Adenomyosis 5, 9, 29, 31
Adrenal hyperplasia, congenital 5, 28
Adrenal tumor 5
Adrenaline 209
Amenorrhea, lactational 24
Amniocentesis 85, 89
Amniotic fluid
- embolism 107, 117, 123, 143, 149
- index 198

Ampicillin 105, 208
Anaerobes 209
Anaphylaxis 107
- treatment of 209

Androgen insensitivity syndrome 27
Android 213
Anencephaly 90, 200
Anesthesia 16
Angiotensin-converting enzyme inhibitor 97, 207
Anomaly ultrasound scan 85, 130
Antenatal care 85, 157
Anthropoid 213
Antibiotics 76
Antibody 85, 198
Anticholinergics 23
Anticoagulation 145
Antidepressants 106, 142
Antihypertensives 136
Anti-Müllerian hormone, absence of 222
Antiphospholipid syndrome 108
Anxiolytics therapy 106
Aortic dissection 107
Aortic root dissecting aneurysm 139
Appendicitis 9, 112, 145, 212
Arterial blood gases 101, 110
Asherman syndrome 6, 30
Aspirin 102, 111, 138, 203, 205
Assisted vaginal breech delivery 92, 118, 150
Asthma 100, 205
- controlled 205
- mild 205

Atypia 16, 34
Autoimmune condition 76
Autosomal dominant inheritance 128, 155
Autosomal recessive
- conditions 221
- inheritance 128, 155

B

Bacterial vaginosis 11, 14, 33
Bacteriuria, asymptomatic 206
Bakri balloon 122, 151
Bartholin's abscesses 76
Bartholomew's rule 85, 130
Benzathine penicillin 32, 76, 208
Biophysical score 199
Biopsy
- cone 15, 34
- directed 13
- endometrial 72, 77
- pipelle 17

Bishop's score 213
Bladder 68
- retraining 23, 38
- ultrasound scan of 37

Bleeding, vaginal 82, 144
Blood
- culture 209, 219
- group 84, 210
- loss 215, 217
- pressure 131
- stained discharge 126, 218
- volume 198

Body mass index 87, 131

Botulinum toxin 23
Bowel 68
obstruction 112
Brace suture 122
Brachytherapy 34
Breast
abscess 125, 126
cancer 126
engorgement 126
lump 126
Brenner tumor 10
Bronchopneumonia 100, 125, 138
Bronchoscopy 101
Burch colposuspension 25

C

Cancer
breast 126
endometrial 16, 56
ovarian 17, 57
vaginal 18, 58
vulva 18, 58
Candida albicans 11, 13
Carcinoma
mixed 16
vulva 20
Cardiac echo 132
Cardiac output 131
Cardinal ligament 27
Cardiomyopathy 107
types of 206
Cardiotocography 88
Ceftriaxone 32
Cephalic 201
Cervical cancer 55, 77, 82, 93
Cervical cerclage 109, 143
removal of 144
Cervical cytology 19
Cervical ectopy 93
Cervical ectropion 30
Cervical edema 215
Cervical length measurement 85
Cervical tear 117, 121, 151
Cervicitis 93
Cesarean section 25
Chemoradiation 15, 20
Chemotherapy 15, 20, 78
adjuvant 20, 36
neoadjuvant 20
Chest X-ray 138
Chickenpox 104, 140, 207
Chills 221
Chlamydia
screening 7
trachomatis 11, 14, 32, 75, 104, 141, 208
Cholecystitis, acute 112, 146
Chorioamnionitis 108, 112, 146, 152
Chronic renal disease 87, 94, 131
Clear cell carcinoma 16
Clostridium perfringens 219
Clot dysmenorrhea 72
Coagulation
disorder 5
factors 198
Cocaine 87
Colpocleisis 24, 38
Colposcopy 13, 19, 33
Combined contraceptive pill 24, 38
Combined hormonal contraceptive 6, 31, 70, 74, 78, 82
patch 24
ring 24, 38
Complete blood count 72
Complete molar pregnancy 28, 70
Constipation 45
Contraception 24, 63
Copper intrauterine device 24, 83
Cord
entanglement 91, 133
prolapse 147
Cordocentesis 89
Coronavirus disease-2019 100, 104, 141, 207
Corticosteroids 92, 109, 133, 143, 211
Couvelaire uterus 117, 149, 202
Cow's milk 219
C-reactive protein 125
Crown rump length 85, 198
Cryotherapy 13
Crystalline penicillin 105, 141, 208
Culture 130
endocervical swab for 12
Cusco's speculum 27
Cushing's syndrome 5, 137
Cyclical progestogens 6
Cyclizine 71
Cystadenocarcinoma, serous 17, 35
Cystadenoma, serous 10
Cystic fibrosis 100, 205
Cystic hygroma 90

Cystocele 80
Cystoscopy 25
Cytomegalovirus 104, 207

D

Dark-field microscopy 12
Deep vein thrombosis 25
Degenerating fibroid 146, 212
Dehydration 71
Deinfibulation
  intrapartum 127
  postdelivery 127
Depression, postpartum 209
Dermatitis 13, 33
Dermoid 74
  ovarian cyst 10, 32
Diabetes mellitus 5, 204
  gestational 87, 108, 143, 204
  monitoring of 203
Dichorionic 200
Dietary modification 70, 203
Direct maternal mortality 154
Disseminated intravascular coagulation 117
Dorsal position 68
Down syndrome 200
Drug toxicity 142
Ductus venosus, Doppler of 88
Duloxetine 23, 38
Duodenal atresia 87, 90, 131
Dysfunctional uterine contractions 215
Dysgerminoma 17
Dysmenorrhea, primary 9, 31

E

Echogenic bowel 200
Eclampsia 94, 135
Edward syndrome 200
Electroconvulsive therapy 106
Electrolyte 69
  disturbance 71
Embryology, basic 40
Endocrine carcinoma 16
Endodermal sinus tumor 17
Endometrial pathology 5
Endometrioid cystadenocarcinoma 17
Endometrioma 10, 74
Endometriosis 9, 31, 50, 76
Endometritis 123, 125, 152
Epidural catheter 145
Epigastric artery, inferior 39
Episiotomy 121, 189
Epithelial ovarian cancers 79
Ergometrine 122, 205
Erythroid progenitor cells 208
Erythromycin 109
Escherichia coli 206, 219
Estradiol 31
Estradiol levels 69
Estrogen 21, 36
Ethambutol 142
Exomphalos 90, 132

F

Fallopian tube cancer 17, 57
Fasting blood glucose 98, 137
Female genital mutilation 127, 194
Fetal blood sample 116, 118, 119, 148, 149
Fetal growth 87, 158
  restriction 199, 204
  ultrasound 96, 131, 135
Fetal heart motion, absence of 210
Fetal kick chart 88
Fetal kidneys 198
Fetal membranes
  artificial rupture of 146
  premature rupture of 109, 177
Fetal monitoring 87, 158
Fibroids 5
Fibroma 10, 126
Flexion point 216
Flucloxacillin 220
Fluids 149
Fluoxetine 21
Folic acid 136, 140
Follicle-stimulating hormone 2
Follicular cyst 10, 32
Fortuitous maternal death 154
Fourth-generation test 12
Free fetal deoxyribonucleic acid 211
Functional ovarian cyst 10, 32

G

Gardnerella vaginalis 14
Gastroschisis 90, 133
Genital herpes 209
Genital prolapse 22, 61

Genital tract
premalignant disorders of 13, 54
trauma 152
Genotype, cord blood for 212
Germ cells migrate 222
Gestation, weeks of 201
Gestational age 198
Gestational diabetes 87, 108, 143, 204
diagnosis of 203
risk factors for 197
Glomeruloendotheliosis 94
Glucose tolerance test 85, 130, 137
Gonadotropin-releasing hormone antagonist 31
Granulosa cell tumor 10, 17, 35
Grave's diseases 204
Gravidity 85
Group B hemolytic streptococcus 104
Growth scan 105
Gynecoid 213
Gynecological oncology 15, 55
Gynecology 1
applied genetics in 128
history 1, 41
physical examination 1, 41
principles of surgery in 25, 65

H

Haemophilus influenzae 14
infection 138
Head, delivery of 216
Heart 211
block 205
disease 205
failure, anemic 208
rate, fetal 147, 199
HELLP syndrome 94, 135
Hematocolpos 71
Hematometra 71
Hemoglobin genotype 85
Hemophilia A 222
Hemorrhage 79, 84, 107, 199, 209, 220
antepartum 93, 163
intrapartum 199
postpartum 122, 189
Hemorrhagic corpus luteum cyst 10
Heparin, unfractionated 144
Hepatitis 11, 104
virus 207
Hernia
diaphragmatic 90, 132
hiatus 112
Herpes
genitalis 141
simplex 11, 13, 32, 141
infection, diagnosis of 207
virus 75, 175
Histology, biopsy for 19, 36
Hormone replacement therapy 21, 59
Human chorionic gonadotropin 199
Human immunodeficiency virus 11, 141
Human papillomaviruses 11, 75
Hydralazine 95
Hyperplasia, endometrial 16, 34
Hyperprolactinemia 6
Hypertension 203
essential 94, 135
pregnancy-induced 135
Hyperthyroidism 137
Hypnotism 21
Hypoglycemia 107
Hypothyroidism 5, 29, 108, 137
Hysterectomy 6, 13, 29, 78, 122, 152
total abdominal 78
vaginal 24
Hysterosalpingography 7, 30

I

Ichthyosis 99
Imipramine 106
Immunoglobulin 219
G 175
M 175
Imperforate hymen 68, 71
Infection 152
fetal 87
Infertility treatment 206
Influenza 100, 104
Infracolic omentectomy 78
Inhibin 69
Instrumental delivery 124, 148, 206, 217
Insulin 98, 136
Internal artery ligation, bilateral 122
Internal iliac, anterior division of 27
Interstitial cystitis 9
Interstitial portion 68
Intrahepatic cholestasis 99
Intrauterine adhesions 6, 30

Intrauterine balloon tamponade 122, 151
Intrauterine devices 81
Intrauterine fetal death 108, 133, 176
Ipsilateral lymph node dissection 36
Iron deficiency 211
Irritable bowel syndrome 9
Isoniazid 105, 141
Itching 76

J

Juvenile diabetes, increase risk of 219

K

Karyotype 7
Kidneys 37
Kleihauer test 4
Klinefelter syndrome 6

L

Labetalol 95, 135, 203
Labia
  inspection of 68
  minora 220
Labor 112, 145
  abnormal 117, 186
  induction of 95, 105, 109, 113, 119, 124, 134, 182
  lasting 216
  latent phase of 147
  normal 114, 183
  progress of 147
Lactation 126, 192
Laparoscopy, diagnostic 74, 39
Laparotomy 113
Legs, compression duplex Doppler of 144
Leiomyoma 5, 73
Leopold's maneuvers 85, 130
Lethal fetomaternal hemorrhage 108, 143
Levonorgestrel intrauterine system 6, 30, 82
Lichen
  planus 13
  sclerosus 13, 33
Listeria monocytogenes 104
Lithium carbonate 106
Liver
  disease, active 80
  enzymes, elevated 203
Lobar pneumonia 100, 125, 138, 153, 205
Lochia
  alba 218
  rubra 218
  serosa 218
Low molecular weight heparin 145, 205
  dose of 145
Low-lying placenta 93, 134
Lumbar 83
Lung
  collapse 100
  disease, suppurative 100

M

Macrosomia, Fetal 124
Magnesium sulfate 95, 107, 109, 135, 143
Malaria 104, 141
Malformations, congenital 199, 204
Malignancy 5
Marfan syndrome 139, 206
Marsupialization 76
Mastitis 125, 126, 154
Maternal death, direct cause of 220
Maternal mortality 85, 127, 194
  direct 131
  indirect 131, 154
Mathew Duncan's technique 116
Mefenamic acid 6
Meigs syndrome 79
Membranes 218
  artificial rupture of 113, 213
  retained 123, 152
Meningitis 125
Menopause 21, 59
  onset of 80
Menstrual period, last 3
Menstruation
  disorders of 5, 42, 46
  physiology 42
Metformin 98, 136
  prepregnancy dose of 137
Methotrexate 28
Methyldopa 95
Middle cerebral artery Doppler 96
Miscarriage 5, 204
  complete 28
  inevitable 28
  spontaneous 199
  threatened 69

Misoprostol 122
Mitochondrial inheritance 128
Moisturizers 21
Monochorionic twins 200
Monozygotic 200
Mosaicism 128, 155
  increased risk of 200
Mucinous cystadenocarcinoma 17
Mucinous cystadenoma 10
Müllerian agenesis 69
Müllerian ducts 222
Multifactorial inheritance 128
Mumps orchitis 6
Myocardial infarction 107, 139, 142
Myomectomy 6, 39
Myometrium, sarcoma of 16

N

Naegele's rule 85, 197
Nausea 45
Neisseria gonorrhoeae 11, 14, 75, 76, 104, 141
Neonatal death 85
  early 154, 220
  rate 88, 131
Neonatal respiratory depression, increased risk of 215
Nephrotic syndrome 94
Neurofibromatosis 5
Nexplanon 38, 82
Nifedipine 95, 211
Nipple
  cracked 126
  retracted 126, 153
Noninvasive prenatal testing 132
Nontreponemal test 12, 32
Norethindrone 31
Nuchal fold 199
Nuchal translucency measurement 85
Nucleic acid amplification test 12, 32

O

Obesity, maternal 124, 131, 152
Obstetric 85
  applied genetics in 128, 196
  cholestasis 108, 215
  examination 85, 156
  history 85, 156
Outflow obstruction 22
Ovarian cyst 9
Ovarian cystectomy 31
Ovarian disorders, benign 10, 51
Ovarian estrogen 69
Ovarian torsion 74, 112
Ovarian tumor, estrogen-producing 5, 29
Ovarian vein 27, 39
Overactive bladder 22, 37
Oxygen saturation 215
Oxytocin 206

P

Paget's disease 13
Pains, sudden-onset abdominal 148
Palliative care 20
Pancreatitis, acute 112, 146
Paracetamol 149
Parity 85, 130
Parvovirus B19 104, 140, 207
Pelvic brim 197, 214
Pelvic floor exercises 23, 38, 81
Pelvic inflammatory disease, acute 9
Pelvic organ 218
Pelvic pain, chronic 9, 50
Pelvis
  contracted 213
  MRI of 36
  types of 213
Pemphigoid gestationis 99, 137, 204
Penicillin G 208
Peptic ulcer disease 112
Perinatal death 85
Perinatal mortality 85, 127, 194
  rate 88, 131
Perineal pain 218
Perineal tear 121, 189
  first-degree 121
  fourth-degree 121, 217
  third degree 151, 217
Periurethral tear 121
Pessary, right 24
Placenta 218
  accreta 93
  delivery of 218
  percreta 93, 134
  previa 124
  retained 123

Placental abruption 93, 112, 123, 134, 202
Placental migration 201
Placental previa 93, 202
Plasma fibrinogen levels 198
Platelet
 count 131
 low 203
Platypelloid 213
Pleural effusion 100
Polycystic ovary syndrome 5, 72
Polygenic inheritance 128
Polyhydramnios 124, 202, 203
Polymerase chain reaction, bronchial lavage for 138
Positron emission tomography scan 36
Pre-eclampsia 94
Pregnancy 198, 205
 abdominal pain in 112, 181
 assessment unit, early 4
 atopic eruption of 99, 138, 204
 bleeding in 93, 163
 cardiac disorders in 102, 170
 complications 3, 43, 204
 connective tissue disorder of 102, 169
 dermatological disorders of 99, 167
 ectopic 70
 endocrine disorders of 97, 99, 166, 167
 gastrointestinal disorders in 45
 hematological disorders of 110, 179
 hypertensive disorders of 94, 165, 202
 hypothyroidism in 204
 infections in 104, 172
 maternal collapse in 107, 176
 multiple 91, 124, 152, 162, 200
 normal physiology of 86, 158
 polymorphic eruption of 99, 137, 204
 psychiatric disorders in 106, 175
 renal disorders of 103, 171
 respiratory disorders of 100, 168
 total number of 197
 trimesters 130
 viral infection in 140, 207
Prenatal diagnosis 89
 management 160
Preterm 216
 delivery 201, 210, 221
 labor 109, 177, 204
Primigravida 94
Progesterone, low 69
Progestogen 21, 36, 106
Prostaglandin 218
 pessaries 114
Protein A 212
Proteinuria 206
Psoriasis 13, 99
Psychiatric assessment 154
Psychotherapy 106, 142
Pubertal disorders 2, 5, 41, 45
Puberty 2, 5, 41, 45
Puerperal disorders 125, 191
Puerperium disorders 125, 191
Pulmonary embolism 100, 125, 153
Pulmonary stenosis 139
Pulse oximetry 110, 138
Punch biopsy 77
Pyelonephritis 112, 125, 146, 153
Pyrazinamide 142

Q

Quadruple test 85

R

Radical hysterectomy 15, 34
Radical vulvectomy 20
Radical wide excision 36
Radiotherapy 20, 36
 external 34
Rectocele 80
Rectovaginal fistula 121
Reflexology 21
Reflux esophagitis 112
Renal assessment 136
Renal failure 77, 94
Renal function 206
Renal ultrasound scan 103, 139
Reproduction, basic anatomy and physiology of 40
Retinal assessment 136
Rhesus isoimmunization 108
Ribonucleic acid 207
Rifampicin 105, 141
Rosacea 99
Rub uterine contractions 122, 151, 218
Rubella 104

S

Sacrocolpopexy 24, 39
Sacrospinous fixation 24, 80
Salpingo-oophorectomy, bilateral 78
Sampson, implantation theory of 74
Sarcoma botryoides 79
Scabies 99
Scaphoid 213
Seborrheic dermatitis 99
Selective fetal growth restriction 91, 133
Semen analysis 7, 30
Sensitivity 130
  endocervical swab for 12
Sepsis 84, 142
Sertoli-Leydig tumor 17, 35
Serum prolactin 7, 30
Sex-determining region 68, 222
Sex-linked recessive
  disorders 222
  inheritance 128, 155
Sexually transmitted infections 11, 52, 84, 207
Sheehan's syndrome 6
Sims speculum 27
Speculum examination 29, 143, 211
Spina bifida 132
Spiral artery, abnormal trophoblastic invasion of 202
Spontaneous preterm labor 221
Squamous cell carcinoma 16, 79
Sterilization 39
Stillbirth 88
  number of 199
  rate 131
Streptococcus pyogenes 14
Streptomycin 105, 142, 208
Subdermal implant 38, 82
Subfertility 6, 48
Suboccipito-bregmatic 216
Supportive therapy 106
Sweating 221
Symphysis pubic dysfunction 112
Syntocinon 122, 148
  augmentation 124, 152
  infusion 154
Syntometrine 122, 151
Syphilis 75, 104, 140
Systemic lupus erythematosus, complication of 143

T

Tachycardia, fetal 125
Tachysystole 113
Tension pneumothorax 100, 107, 138
Teratoma, immature 17
Terbutaline 146, 150
Testosterone implants 21
Thrombocytopenia 117
Thromboprophylaxis 205, 206
Thyroid-stimulating hormone receptor antibodies 204
Thyrotoxicosis 204
Tocolysis 109, 143, 211
Tongue, under surface of 197
Tonsillitis 125
Toxicity 107
Toxoplasma gondii 104, 140
Toxoplasmosis 208
Trachelectomy 15
Tranexamic acid 6, 122
Transabdominal ultrasound scan 27
Transient tachypnea, increased risk of 217
Transvaginal ultrasound scan 7, 29, 70, 134
Transverse cervical ligament 80
Treponema pallidum 140
  hemagglutination assay 208
Treponemal test 12
Trichomonas vaginalis 11, 14, 33
Tricyclic antidepressant 106
T-sign 201
Tubal disease 6, 30
Tubal patency test 30
Tuberculosis 140
  pulmonary 140
Tubo-ovarian mass 10
Tubular necrosis 94
Tumor 69
Turner syndrome, clinical features of 69
Twin growth, normal discordant 133
Twin reversal arterial perfusion sequence 91
Twin-peak sign, absence of 200
Twin-to-twin transfusion
  stage 91
  syndrome 133, 201

U

Ultrasound scan 85, 198
Umbilical artery 199
  Doppler 88, 96, 135
Urea 69
Ureteric colic 112
Ureters 37
Urethral swabs 27
Uric acid 96
Urinalysis 37, 81, 85, 95, 96, 136, 211
Urinary fistula 22
Urinary incontinence, mixed 22, 37
Urinary tract infection 125, 153
Urine
  collection, twenty-four hours 96
  microscopy 130
  pregnancy test 74
  protein creatinine ratio 202
  spot polymerase chain reaction 136
  spot protein-creatinine ratio 96
Urodynamic stress incontinence 22, 37
Urogynecology 22, 61
Uterine
  artery 1, 39
    Doppler 96
    embolization 6
  atony 117, 152, 217
  bleeding, abnormal 5, 46
  fibroids 9, 31, 72, 124
  fundus 214
  hyperstimulation 113
  inversion 117, 149, 218
  rupture 113, 117, 148
Uterus
  benign conditions of 8, 49
  ruptured 213
  serous carcinoma of 16
  well-contracted 218

V

Vaginal delivery, operative 116, 120, 188
Vaginal orifice, narrowing of 220
Vaginal tear 151
Vaginectomy, total 20
Vague symptoms 78
Varicella zoster 207
  immunoglobulin 142
Varicose veins 93
Vas, congenital absence of 6, 30
Vasa previa 93
  diagnosis of 134, 202
Venous thromboembolism 153
Ventilation perfusion 110
Viral polymerase chain reaction, fluid for 32, 207
Vitiligo 99
Vomiting 45
Vulva
  benign conditions of 13, 54
  eczema 33
Vulvodynia 13, 33
Vulvovaginal candidiasis 14, 33

W

Warfarin sodium 111
Weight loss 71
Wertheim's hysterectomy 15, 34
Wound infection 125

Y

Y chromosome 68, 222
Yolk sac 222

Z

Ziehl-Neelsen staining 140
Zika virus 104